Cancer Risks

Strategies for Elimination

Edited by
Peter Bannasch

With 34 Figures

Springer-Verlag
Berlin Heidelberg New York
London Paris Tokyo

Prof. Dr. PETER BANNASCH
Institut für Experimentelle Pathologie
Deutsches Krebsforschungszentrum
Im Neuenheimer Feld 280
D-6900 Heidelberg

The publication of this book was supported by the Arbeitsgemeinschaft für Grossforschungseinrichtungen (AGF).

Institutions participating in the AGF-Koordinierungsausschuß Krebsforschung

DKFZ Deutsches Krebsforschungszentrum Heidelberg
GBF Gesellschaft für Biotechnologische Forschung Braunschweig
GSF Gesellschaft für Strahlen- und Umweltforschung Neuherberg
KFA Kernforschungsanlage Jülich
KfK Kernforschungszentrum Karlsruhe

Library of Congress Cataloging-in-Publication Data. Cancer risks. Includes bibliographies and index. 1. Cancer – Prevention. 2. Carcinogens. 3. Carcinogenesis. 4. Health risk assessment. I. Bannasch, Peter. [DNLM: 1. Carcinogens – toxicity. 2. Neoplasms – prevention & control. 3. Oncogenic Viruses – pathogenicity. QZ 202 C21564]
RC268.C3676 1987 616.99'4052 87-4350
ISBN-13: 978-3-540-17465-3 e-ISBN-13: 978-3-642-71843-4
DOI: 10.1007/ 978-3-642-71843-4

Typesetting by, Petersche Druckerei GmbH & Co. Offset KG, Rothenburg ob der Tauber
2121/3130-543210

Preface

A large body of information about possible causes of cancer has been accumulated by both clinical experience in man and observations in animal experiments. There is general agreement that in most cases cancer is due to exogenous factors, albeit the genetic disposition may also play an important part. Three main categories of exogenous risk factors have been identified, namely chemicals, radiation, and viruses. In principle, it should be possible to prevent cancer by eliminating such risk factors. However, in spite of the rapidly growing number of well established risk factors, many shortcomings in our understanding of the causes of human cancer and in the introduction of effective preventive measures are evident. In addition to obvious gaps in our scientific knowledge, inadequacies in personal life style, irresponsible handling of environmental contaminants, and in some areas also deficiencies in political decisions seriously hamper the elimination of risk factors for cancer.

It was this background which prompted the Committee coordinating Cancer Research in the Großforschungseinrichtungen in the Federal Republic of Germany to organize a conference on Strategies for the Elimination of Cancer Risks. The conference was held in Heidelberg in June 1986. In areas which appeared to be especially pertinent to public health, authoritative speakers presented the state of the art and prepared the basis for the discussion. Both the presentations of the speakers and the summaries of the discussions are contained in this book.

The idea of the conference emerged long before the atomic energy plant accident in Chernobyl and the severe chemical pollution of the river Rhine had happened. Some of the consequences of the Chernobyl accident were discussed at the conference. As to the chemical risk factors, in addition to occupational cancer, special emphasis was laid upon tobacco smoking, one of the best known risk factors for cancer in man. The discussion on viruses as possible risk factors for human cancer aims at the development of vaccines which might prevent certain types of cancer.

I am obliged to all members of the Scientific Committee who gave valuable advice for the program of the conference: L. E. Feinendegen (Düsseldorf/Jülich), W. Gössner (Munich), U. Hagen (Munich/Neuherberg), H. zur Hausen (Heidelberg), P. Herrlich (Karlsruhe), P. Mühlradt (Braunschweig), R. Preussmann (Heidelberg), and D. Schmähl (Heidelberg). I am also grateful to the Administration of the German Cancer Research Center and to my coworkers, who guaranteed a smooth running of the meeting. My special thanks go to the speakers, the moderators, and the rapporteurs of the discussions, and to all the participants who contributed to the success of the meeting and provided the basis for this book. Finally, I am indebted to Ute Heilmann of Springer-Verlag for excellent cooperation and much support in achieving rapid publication of the proceedings.

Heidelberg, December 5, 1986 PETER BANNASCH

Contents

Session 3
Chemical Carcinogens: Primary Prevention
Chairman: D. SCHMÄHL

Session 4
Physical Carcinogens
Chairman: W. GÖSSNER

Session 5
Oncogenic Viruses
Chairman: E. WECKER

List of Contributors

ANDRAE, ULRICH, Institut für Toxikologie der Gesellschaft für Strahlen- und Umweltforschung, D-8042 Neuherberg, FRG

ARAB-KOHLMEIER, LENORE, Bundesgesundheitsamt, Institut für Sozialmedizin und Epidemiologie, Postfach 330013, D-1000 Berlin 33, FRG

BANNASCH, PETER, Institut für Experimentelle Pathologie, Deutsches Krebsforschungszentrum, Im Neuenheimer Feld 280, D-6900 Heidelberg, FRG

BASS, ROLF, Bundesgesundheitsamt, Thielallee 88–92, D-1000 Berlin 33, FRG

BRUNNEMANN, KLAUS D., Naylor Dana Institute for Disease Prevention, American Health Foundation, Valhalla, NY 10595, U.S.A.

DEINHARDT, FRIEDRICH, Max von Pettenkofer Institut für Hygiene und Medizinische Mikrobiologie der Ludwig-Maximilians-Universität München, Pettenkoferstr. 9, D-8000 München 2, FRG

DOLL, RICHARD, SIR, Imperial Cancer Research Fund, Cancer Epidemiology Unit, Radcliffe Infirmary, Oxford OX2 6HE, U.K.

EISENBRAND, GERHARD, Lebensmittelchemie und Umwelttoxikologie der Universität Kaiserslautern, Erwin-Schrödinger-Str., D-6750 Kaiserslautern, FRG

ENZMANN, HARALD, Institut für Experimentelle Pathologie, Deutsches Krebsforschungszentrum, Im Neuenheimer Feld 280, D-6900 Heidelberg, FRG

GÖGGELMANN, WALTRAUD, Institut für Toxikologie der Gesellschaft für Strahlen- und Umweltforschung, D-8042 Neuherberg, FRG

GREIM, HELMUT, Institut für Toxikologie der Gesellschaft für Strahlen- und Umweltforschung, D-8042 Neuherberg, FRG

HAHN, ERIC W., Institut für Nuklearmedizin, Deutsches Krebsforschungszentrum, Im Neuenheimer Feld 280, D-6900 Heidelberg, FRG

HALEY, NANCY J., Naylor Dana Institute for Disease Prevention, American Health Foundation, Valhalla, NY 10595, U.S.A.

HARNDEN, DAVID G., The Paterson Laboratories, Christie Hospital and Holt Radium Institute, Wilmslow Road, Manchester M20 9BX, U.K.

HAUSEN ZUR, HARALD, Deutsches Krebsforschungszentrum, Im Neuenheimer Feld 280, D-6900 Heidelberg, FRG

HECHT, STEPHEN S., Naylor Dana Institute for Disease Prevention, American Health Foundation, Valhalla, NY 10595, U.S.A.

HENSCHLER, DIETER, Institut für Pharmakologie und Toxikologie, Universität Würzburg, Versbacher Landstr. 9, D-8700 Würzburg, FRG

HOFFMANN, DIETRICH, Naylor Dana Institute for Disease Prevention, American Health Foundation, Valhalla, NY 10595, U.S.A.

HUNSMANN, GERHARD, Abteilung für Virologie und Immunologie, Deutsches Primatenzentrum, Kellnerweg 4, D-3400 Göttingen, FRG

IPPEN, HELMUT, Abt. Dermatologie und Venerologie I, Universitäts-Hautklinik, von Siebold-Str. 3, D-3400 Göttingen, FRG

JAKOBI, WOLFGANG, GSF Neuherberg, Institut für Strahlenschutz, Ingolstädter Landstr. 1, D-8042 Neuherberg, FRG

KELLERER, ALBRECHT M., Institut für Medizinische Strahlenkunde, Universität Würzburg, Versbacher Landstr. 5, D-8700 Würzburg, FRG

LANDRIGAN, PHILIPP J., Environmental Sciences Laboratory, Mount Sinai School of Medicine of The City of New York, 10 East 102nd Street, New York, NY 10029, U.S.A.

LAVOIE, EDMOND J., Naylor Dana Institute for Disease Prevention, American Health Foundation, Valhalla, NY 10595, U.S.A.

NEUMANN, HANS-GÜNTER, Institut für Pharmakologie und Toxikologie, Universität Würzburg, Versbacher Landstr. 9, D-8700 Würzburg, FRG

ORLANDI, MARIO A., American Health Foundation, 320 East 43rd Street, New York, NY 10017, U.S.A.

PREUSSMANN, RUDOLF, Institut für Toxikologie und Chemotherapie, Deutsches Krebsforschungszentrum, Im Neuenheimer Feld 280, D-6900 Heidelberg, FRG

PURCHASE, IAIN F. H., Central Toxicology Laboratory, Imperial Chemical Institutes PLC., Alderley Park near Macclesfield, Chesire SK10 4TJ, U.K.

SCHWARZ, LESLIE, Institut für Toxikologie der Gesellschaft für Strahlen- und Umweltforschung, D-8042 Neuherberg, FRG

SELIKOFF, IRVING J., Environmental Sciences Laboratory, Mount Sinai School of Medicine of The City University of New York, 10 East 102nd Street, New York, NY 10029, U.S.A.

SUMMER, KARL-HEINZ, Institut für Toxikologie der Gesellschaft für Strahlen- und Umweltforschung, D-8042 Neuherberg, FRG

WYNDER, ERNEST L., American Health Foundation, Mahoney Institute Maintenance, 320 East 43rd Street, New York, NY 10017, U.S.A.

ZERBAN, HEIDE, Institut für Experimentelle Pathologie, Deutsches Krebsforschungszentrum, Im Neuenheimer Feld 280, D-6900 Heidelberg, FRG

SESSION 1

General Aspects

Chairman: F. Vogel

Genetic Predisposition for Cancer Risks in Man

D. G. Harnden

General Introduction

In considering cancer risks and strategies for their elimination it is vitally important to keep in mind the diverse nature of the disease. Not only are there many different kinds of cancer, each with subtypes, but also it seems likely that for any one cancer there may be a variety of interacting causal factors. Moreover, there is good evidence that the same cancer type may be the end result of a number of quite different causal pathways. Such considerations will have both advantages and disadvantages in trying to understand cancer. On the negative side, the sheer complexity of the causal mechanisms makes both analysis of the aetiology and proposals for preventive action extremely difficult and, of course, the existence of multiple pathways can mean that even a successful strategy may not deal adequately with all the risks. On the other hand our growing power to resolve subclasses of disease often means that we can see a causal pattern clearly for the first time even though the number of cases in that category may be small. Furthermore, the existence of multiple factors in the aetiology of a cancer, while it may make complete elucidation of mechanisms difficult, means that removal of only one of the causal factors may make a major impact in reducing incidence even in the absence of complete understanding.

The place of genetic factors in cancer risk must be seen within this context. It is likely that inherited risk will be only one component in many in considering the causation of most cancers. It may be very important in some cancers, but relatively unimportant in others. It may be a factor in only some subtypes and, within any one cancer, it may be a factor for some cases but not for others. But, as far as risk elimination is concerned, knowledge of the genetic element may be vitally important since, if we can identify those at risk and separate them or protect them in some way from the other interacting factors, risk reduction may be achieved in cases where such protection would be difficult by other means.

Genetic/Environmental Interactions

Many environmental factors involved in the causation of cancer have been identified and these will be dealt with in detail by Sir Richard Doll in the next presentation. It is also well established that many factors intrinsic to the patient are important in determining cancer incidence. Amongst these are age, hormone balance, capacity for immune response and genetic constitution. These extrinsic and intrinsic factors will interact with each other. For example, it is clear that there is a close interrelationship between oncogenic viruses and the ability of the subject to mount an immune response. The effect of oncogenic viruses is also age dependent. Similarly, the carcinogenic effect of radiation exposure is influenced both by age and by genetic constitution. Nevertheless, much evidence points to the very powerful influence of environmental factors in many situations and also to the difficulty of demonstrating convincingly a genetic component in the common cancers. It is quite usual, therefore, to ascribe a certain proportion of cancer to "the environment". How the others are caused is left unsaid. It is clearly inappropriate, however, to imagine that, say 80% of cancers are due to environmental causes, while 20% are due to genetic factors. We must change this way of thinking entirely and regard environmental factors as likely to be involved as causal agents in all cancers. These environmental agents will, however, be acting on a population of great diversity and the response of an individual will depend not only upon the strength of the environmental influence but also upon the way in which that environmental stimulus is handled by the individual and upon the way in which any altered cells are handled by systemic influences within the body of that individual. Much of this variation in response will be genetic in origin and it is, therefore, equally true to say that all cancers will be influenced by genetic factors. Obviously if the environmental exposure is overwhelming there will be little observable impact of the genetic element. What we must seek to understand therefore, is the relative importance of environmental factors and of hereditary influences in the development of particular cancers. It is probable that in many instances the environmental component is the more important, but if we are to understand the mode of action of environmental agents we must take into consideration the variability in the population upon which those agents are operating.

It is necessary to consider, in this context, why it is that genetic effects are not immediately apparent if, indeed, they are as important as I am suggesting. There are two points to consider. First, where we are looking for a genetic/environmental interaction we would not expect to recognize cancer susceptibility as a simple Mendelian trait unless (a) the probability of encountering the necessary environmental stimulus, (b) the probability of the critical interaction occurring at the cellular level and (c) the probability of the altered cells progressing to a clinical cancer are all close to 100%. Second, if there is a substantial group in the population susceptible to the carcinogenic effects of a rare environmental event it might be hard to define that group unless there were another marker for susceptibility. A genetic factor could be operating and yet be unrecognized because we do not know what it is that we are looking for. We are aware of many genetic polymorphisms in the population only because we have sophisticated tools for recognizing them at our disposal. For example, if we did not have typing sera, blood groups would be unrecognized but they would still exist. If we did not have gel electrophoresis techniques, enzyme polymorphisms would not disappear overnight but we could not see them. Similarly, substantial genetic polymorphisms conferring susceptibility to cancer could exist unrecognized within the population. This problem is one aspect of the problem of "penetrance" of cancer susceptibility genes. If a gene has low penetrance for whatever reason, a genetic effect would not be easy to detect.

Mechanisms by which Genetically Determined Cancer Susceptibility Might Operate

Cancer susceptibility may operate at several different levels regardless of the mode of inheritance.

Direct Inheritance

First, it is widely agreed that a change, or, more likely a series of changes, in the structure or regulation of the genome of one or more somatic cells are critical steps in the process of carcinogenesis. One possible mechanism of inherited susceptibility is that an individual inherits one of these genomic alterations directly, so that if the other steps follow with normal probability, cancer is more likely to occur. A possible example of such a mechanism occurs in retinoblastoma where Knudson (1971) has suggested a two-mutation model. On the basis of age-incidence curves he has argued that familial cases could be the result of a single somatic mutational step, whereas sporadic cases could result from two sequential somatic mutational steps. While it is possible that some further elaboration of this model might be necessary to fit all the known facts (e.g., an appropriate differentiation step) the basic two-step hypothesis fits well with the recently recognized hemizygozity or apparent homozygozity at the retinoblastoma locus (chromosome 13q14) in retinoblastoma tumour cells. Cavanee et al. (1983, 1985) have demonstrated nondisjunctional chromosome loss, chromosome deletion and somatic recombination at this locus. It seems likely that a child can inherit a gene mutation at this locus and that expression of this abnormal gene is subsequently permitted by deletion of the homologous chromosomal segment. In cases of retinoblastoma where the patient has a constitutional chromosome deletion at 13q14 the second event could be a mutation, so that the order in which the events occur does not appear to matter. In sporadic cases both events would have to be acquired in a single somatic cell and therefore the probability of occurrence is very low.

There are several important consequences of this observation. (a) The retinoblastoma gene which appears to be a dominant gene in families is recessive at the cellular level. Indeed, further consideration shows that all cancer susceptibility genes are likely to be recessive since the expression of such a gene during normal embryogenesis or cellular functioning would inevitably lead to all such cells becoming malignant and this would be incompatible with continuing normal cell functions. (b) This also demonstrates the point previously made that a Mendelian pattern may only be observed if the probability of a second or subsequent event is virtually 100%. (c) Retinoblastoma also appears to be an example of the situation already described where the same end result might arise by two different routes. Furthermore, only one of these has a major hereditary component.

Indirect Effects on Mutation

In some cases what is inherited is not a genetic lesion which is itself involved in the neoplastic process but a gene which by one means or another increases the probability that such an event will occur elsewhere in the cell. For example, in the chromosome breakage syndromes (Fanconi's anaemia, Bloom's syndrome and ataxia-telangiectasia (AT)), the inherited gene appears to be associated with an unusual susceptibility to an environmental agent which increases the probability of specific or non-specific chromosome rearrangements occurring (Ray and German 1981). While the link between these rearrangements and the unusual cancer incidence in these patients is not clear, it is not unreasonable to link the two phenomena. In AT, for example, there is an unusual sensitivity to ionizing radiation which can be demonstrated at clinical, cellular and chromosome levels (Bridges and Harnden 1982). Clones of cytogenetically abnormal T lymphocytes arise and have been shown to proliferate at the expense of their normal counterparts. These clones frequently have highly specific chromosome rearrangements in which the breakpoints have now been shown to be close to loci involved in T-cell differentiation (Kennaugh et al. 1986). In some cases at least the leukaemia which develops in these subjects arises from within the clone with the specific cytogenetic marker (Kaiser-McCaw and Hecht 1982). It seems probable that these acquired rearrangements in this genetically determined disease are akin to the rearrangements which occur in chronic myeloid leukaemia and in the B-cell lymphomas, where specific chromosome rearrangements are associated with modification in proto-oncogene structure and function (de Klein et al. 1982; Taub et al. 1983).

Another perhaps less obvious example of a genetically determined susceptibility to cancer operating through this type of mechanism are those genes which modify the external agent before it interacts with the DNA of the cell. These carcinogen-modifying enzymes have been studied extensively in experimental systems for many years and it is clear that in mice the hydroxylase enzymes which metabolize polycyclic hydrocarbons are under genetic control (Thorgeirsson and Herbert 1977). Claims that inducibility of these systems in man is under the control of a single pair of allelic genes proved to be grossly oversimplified and a mass of confusing data has clouded the issue. However, it is still apparent that considerable heterogeneity exists within the human population for enzymes which activate polycyclic hydrocarbons. How much of this is genetic and how much is acquired is not clear. Nor is there any clear definition of genetic mechanisms, but if we are to understand the mechanisms of chemical carcinogenesis we must also study the variability in metabolism of these compounds. Such concepts are widely accepted in other fields especially the pharmacokinetics of drugs where consideration of variation in the metabolism, persistence and distribution of drugs has become an integral part of the study of the mode of action of these drugs (Sjoqvist 1985).

A third example, so obvious that it is often overlooked, is the role of skin pigmentation in determining the worldwide distribution of squamous- and basal-cell carcinomas of the skin. The incidence of skin cancers in the white population of South Africa is three times that of a comparable population in the UK. The black population, however, get few skin cancers (Waterhouse et al. 1976). The genetically determined skin pigmentation protects the target DNA from the carcinogenic effects of UV irradiation from the sun. This is a classic example of genetic environmental interaction.

Progression

Observations on genetic susceptibility often concentrate on events early in the development of cancer, where an environmental agent is directly interacting with the cell. At this stage genetic influences may be relatively easy to detect. It is also clear, however, that the progression of an initiated cell will be dependent on the response of the body to that potentially neoplastic focus. Factors such as immune response, hormone balance, intercellular communication by growth factors and other stimuli will all control the progression towards cancer or towards elimination. It is clear that such biological parameters must be, to some extent, under genetic control though specific examples of genetic susceptibility to cancer by such mechanisms are not clear-cut. In the immune deficiency syndromes there is good evidence for an increased susceptibility to cancer, especially of lymphoid tissue (Spector et al. 1982). It is likely though not proven that such susceptibility is due at least in part to a failure to recognize and eliminate potentially neoplastic foci. Patients with disorders of sexual development such as Klinefelter's syndrome and XY gonadal dysgenesis are more likely to develop breast cancers and gonadoblastomas, respectively (Harnden et al. 1971; Mulvihill et al. 1975). It is probable that the disturbance of hormone balance in these syndromes plays a part in the development of neoplasia.

Modes of Inheritance

An alternative mode of considering inherited susceptibility to cancer is to look at the way in which such predispositions appear in families and populations.

Mendelian Inheritance

In a large number of different syndromes and conditions, susceptibility to cancer is inherited in a simple Mendelian fashion (McKusick 1983). Numerically, however, these instances account for only a small proportion of the total cases of cancer, since each condition is rare. This is not the place to consider such syndromes in detail. It is sufficient to point out that there are (a) dominant conditions such as polyposis coli, neurofibromatosis, retinoblastoma, multiple endocrine neoplasia type 2 (MEN-2), basal-cell naevus syndrome; (b) recessive diseases such as xerodoma pigmentosa and AT; (c) sex-linked cancer susceptibility conditions such as Duncan's disease (susceptibility to Epstein-Barr virus) and X-linked agammaglobulinaemia. Knowledge of the precise modes of inheritance is vitally important in the management of these families and I will return to that point in a later section.

Chromosomal Abnormalities

A small number of constitutional chromosomal abnormalities are associated with an increased incidence of malignancy. Trisomy 21 (Down's syndrome) is associated with a 10- to 20-fold increased risk of leukaemia in childhood (Miller 1970). Patients with Klinefelter's syndrome (47,XXY) have an increased risk of breast cancer, while females with gonadal dysgenesis are at a very high risk of developing benign or malignant gonadal tumours (Harnden et al. 1971; Mann et al. 1983).

A number of deletion syndromes are associated with subclasses of particular cancers, e.g. about 5% of retinoblastoma patients are found to have a deletion involving chromosome 13q14 (Harnden and Herbert 1982), while patients with Wilm's tumour and the aniridia, genitourinary, retardation syndrome (Wilm's AGR) are found to have deletions of 11p13 (Riccardi et al. 1980)

Cancer Families

There are many well-documented instances of unusually large numbers of cancers occurring in particular families without there being a clear-cut inheritance pattern or a well-defined syndrome (Lynch et al. 1977b). Some of these high-incidence families will be attributable to chance. In a random distribution one could expect a certain degree of clustering, and where that occurs within a single family it will readily come to the attention of those interested in cancer genetics. However, it has now become clear that many instances of familial aggregation cannot be explained away in this manner. In some cases where attention has been drawn to a family where a large number of cases had been recognized, it is found, that the high level of incidence extends into parts of the pedigree which were unknown at the time of the initial observations. Such a finding strengthens the view that this is not a chance finding. Furthermore, when one studies the characteristics of these "familial cases" it is not infrequently found that they differ in some respect from the nonfamilial cases. It may be that there is an earlier age of onset; the prognosis may be different; the probability of spread and the pattern of spread may be different. Thus, there are families in which there is an exceptionally high incidence of carcinoma of the colon, in patients all of whom develop the disease at well below the average age of occurrence for that disease (Lynch et al. 1986). There is also accumulating evidence that in such families the probability of a second primary malignancy occurring is higher than for the normal population. In some cases the familial pattern is close to that expected of a Mendelian trait, but in others there is no clear mode of inheritance. It seems probable that, in these families, the genetic component is one of a number of interacting influences.

Association of Cancer Susceptibility with Normal Traits

Possibly the most important area of all with respect to the development of strategies for prevention is the association of cancer susceptibility with normal characteristics which show variation in the population. Many such associations have been well documented for many years. For example, the link between skin pigmentation, exposure to ultraviolet light and the occurrence of skin cancer, already referred to, extends beyond the simple question of whether or not skin is pigmented or not. The type of melanin is also important so that fair-skinned individuals with red or reddish hair (phaeomelanin) are more likely to be cancer susceptible than those with fair skin and blond hair (eumelanin). Other well-known examples are the association between carcinoma of the stomach and blood group A (McConnell 1966), and between specific combinations of blood groups in the parents (mother A; father O) and the occurrence of choriocarcinoma following pregnancy (Bagshawe et al. 1971). In certain types of leukaemia or lymphoma, specific HLA subtypes are more common (Dausset et al. 1982). Here one has to be cautious about the interpretation since in some cases at least the association may be with survival rather than development of the disease.

More recently, however, the recognition of DNA polymorphisms in the population has opened a whole new field of study. Some of these DNA probes can be multiply polymorphic so that an individual may have a unique pattern (Jeffrey et al. 1985). Attempts are currently being made to link such polymorphisms with particular kinds of cancer.

Other DNA variations are already being used in attempts to recognize individuals with other kinds of genetic disease. In some cases, such as the thalassaemias, the analysis is far advanced while in others, e.g. Duchenne muscular dystrophy, unexpected difficulties have been encountered and the analysis is much more complex than had been anticipated (Kunkel 1986). A number of DNA variations associated with malignant diseases have been reported. For example, Heighway et al. (1986) report a DNA polymorphism close to the c-Ha-ras proto-oncogene on chromosome 11. As originally shown by Krontiris et al. (1985) there are four common alleles of this polymorphism and a large number of rare variants. Krontiris and his colleagues have suggested a link between the rare variants and a variety of malignant diseases. In a more specific study Thein et al. (1986) have found no such association in myelodysplasias. Heighway and his colleagues have studied these polymorphisms in lung cancer patients and they find a quite different frequency of one of the common alleles (a4) in non-small-cell carcinoma of the lung (25%) as compared to small-cell carcinoma of the lung (8%). These figures may be compared to the 15% of the general population who have the a4 allele. While these studies are at an early stage at present they do point the way to possible future studies which could recognize high risk groups within the general population.

Genetic Strategies for Elimination or Limitation of Cancer Risk

Antenatal Diagnosis and Selective Termination of Pregnancy

For several kinds of genetic disease it has already been accepted in many countries that antenatal diagnosis, and the selective termination of those pregnancies where a serious genetic defect is recognized, is a reasonable strategy for reducing the number of retarded or otherwise handicapped individuals in the population. Such screening is most effective where a high risk-group can be recognized, e.g. mothers over 38 years of age have an elevated risk of having a baby with Down's syndrome which may be recognized antenatally by screening amniotic fluid cells for chromosome abnormality. Population screening at much younger ages would be expensive even in cost-benefit terms and might also carry an unacceptably high risk of accidentally induced abortion following amniocentesis. It is already possible to recognize some of the cancer-prone conditions antenatally, especially conditions like xeroderma pigmentosa, Fanconi's anaemia and ataxia telangiectasia (AT) where there is a clear-cut sensitivity to an environmental agent (Ramsay et al. 1974). Similarly the constitutional chromosome abnormalities can already be recognized by sampling either amniotic fluid or chorionic villi.

While no DNA probes are yet available which will confidently recognize any of the cancer susceptibility syndromes, we can anticipate that such probes will be available within the next few years. DNA clones from the 13q14 region have already been developed (Lalande et al. 1984) and several groups are working on the 11p13 region. It is not too early to begin to consider the practical consequence of this new technology. In the case of AT the decisions that would have to be take if antenatal diagnosis becomes routinely available are not too difficult because of the very serious features of this disease – not only the possibility of cancer. Termination would be a realistic option to offer parents. But would it be reasonable for retinoblastoma, where the cure rate is currently over 90% for cases diagnosed early and in the majority of whom the sight can be saved? The problem would become even more difficult if a DNA probe were recognized which enabled identification of susceptibility to a cancer which did not occur until much later in life. We should begin to consider even now the practical and ethical problems that this situation will create.

Early Recognition with Advice on Lifestyle

This approach is already well established for many types of genetic disease. The prototype is phenylketonuria where early recognition by population screening combined with a phenylalanine-free diet prevents the worst manifestations of the disease. There is also a well-proven example in the field of cancer susceptibility. Patients with xeroderma pigmentosum can be recognized very early after birth either by demonstrating UV sensitivity or a defect in excision repair of DNA. If they are protected from sunlight, no skin lesions develop and no skin cancers occur later in life (Lynch et al. 1977a). Although less dramatic than XP we can already give firm advice to people with fair skin – especially the phaeomelanotic (red-haired) type about the importance of avoiding excessive exposure to UV in sunlight. It is not too difficult to envisage other similar situations where particular groups are recognized to have an unusual sensitivity to some component of diet and can be advised to avoid certain foods. Equally it may be possible to recognize groups for whom avoidance of smoking would be of particular importance.

Genetic Screening of Individuals in or Entering High-Risk Situations

Obviously the elimination or minimization of environmental risks should be a primary strategy. However, in some cases decisions are taken which permit certain risks to remain because of the real or perceived benefit to society. If some individuals are at especial hazard if exposed to such a risk they should be protected from it if that is technically possible. Genetic screening for some occupations is well established either to protect the public (red/green colour blindness in train drivers and pilots) or to protect the individual (alpha-1-anti-trypsin deficiency associated with emphysema in wood workers).

I have already mentioned the variation in enzymes which metabolize the polycyclic aromatic hydrocarbons. The screening of individuals in those occupations, e.g. toolsetters where there is a special risk of mineral-oil induced skin cancer, would be feasible even without a firm knowledge of the genetic basis. However, considerable practical difficulties have to be overcome in a situation where the workers know that the cancers acquired in these dirty but high paid jobs can readily be dealt with by radiotherapy.

Recognition of High-Risk Groups for Cancer Screening

Screening methods are available for the early detection of many kinds of cancer, e.g. carcinoma of the uterine cervix, bladder, lung, colon, breast and thyroid. The application of these procedures on a population-wide basis is often difficult to achieve, bearing in mind the competition for health care resources. If, however, high-risk groups can be recognized, it may be possible to achieve cost-effective screening which would not be possible on a population-wide scale. In the most extreme cases this can already be done. In families with polyposis coli, screening of nonaffected but at-risk family members followed by surgery at an appropriate stage in the development of the diseases can dramatically reduce the risk of colonic carcinoma. Similarly, in MEN-2 families, screening, using serum calcitonin levels, is available and surgical treatment at the appropriate time can virtually eliminate the chances of developing a medullary carcinoma of the thyroid (Ponder 1984). Even in cases where there is a strong familial incidence, but no clear inheritance pattern, screening could be most effective. A strong case can be made for breast cancer screening in the relatives of women with a breast cancer occurring at a young age and some evidence of a family history (Mulvihill 1981). The detection rate in such families is likely to be at least 2 or 3 times that in the normal population.

Genetic Counselling

It is vitally important that, when a cancer is recognized that could be familial, an adequate family history is taken and, if appropriate, counselling made available to the family through special genetic advisory centres. Such expert advice can often prevent the occurrence of further cases of cancer in these families but, just as important, it is often possible to reassure members of such families that they are not at risk. The development of at-risk registers for cancer susceptibility, probably oriented towards a specific disease, would help with this aim.

Conclusions

For a relatively small number of situations where there is a genetically determined susceptibility to cancer, techniques are already available on which strategies for risk elimination can be based. It is clear that current developments especially in recombinant DNA technology will lead in the future to new means of recognizing those genetically at risk and hence to the development of new strategies for reduction of cancer risks. Even if we could develop risk elimination methods for all those situations where there is a clear inherited cancer risk, this would probably make only a small impact on the total cancer problem. However, in those situations where genetic factors and environmental factors are interacting but where no clear inheritance pattern is apparent, a study of the variability in the population may lead to the development of strategies, especially the recognition of high-risk groups, which will permit the application of procedures for screening which would not be possible on a population-wide scale. The logical application to risk elimination of our growing knowledge of environmental carcinogens may only be feasible if we take into consideration the variability of the population on which these environmental influences are operating.

References

Bagshawe KD, Rawlings G, Pike MC, Lawler SD (1971) ABO blood groups in trophoblastic neoplasia. Lancet 1:553

Bridges BA, Harnden DG (1982) Ataxia–telangiectasia: a cellular and molecular link between cancer, neuropathology and immune deficiency

Cavanee WK, Dryja TP, Philips RA, Benedict WF, Godbout R, Gallie BL, Murphree AL, Strong LC, White RL (1983) Expression of recessive alleles by chromosomal mechanisms in retinoblastoma. Nature 305:779–784

Cavanee WK, Hansen MF, Nordenskjold M, Kock E, Maumenee I, Squire JA, Philips RA, Gallie BL (1983) Genetic origin of mutations predisposing to retinoblastoma. Science 228:501–503

Dausset J, Colombani J, Hors J (1982) Major histocompatibility complex and cancer with special reference to human familial tumours (Hodgkin's disease and other malignancies). Cancer Surveys 1:119–149

de Klein A, van Kessel AG, Grosveld G, Bartram CR, Hagmeijer A, Bootsma D, Spurr NK, Heisterkamp N, Groffen J, Stephenson JR (1982) A cellular oncogene is translocated to the Philadelphia chromosome in chronic myeloid leukaemia. Nature 300:765–767

Harnden DG, Herbert A (1982) Association of constitutional chromosome rearrangements with neoplasia. Cancer Surveys 1:149–173

Harnden DG, Langlands AO, McLean N (1971) Carcinoma of the breast and Klinefelter's syndrome. J Med Genet 8:460–461

Heighway J, Thatcher N, Cerny T, Hasleton PS (1986) Genetic predispostion to human lung cancer. Br J Cancer 53:453–457

Jeffreys A, Brookfield JFY, Semeonoff R (1985) Positive identification of an immigration test-case using human DNA fingerprints. Nature 317:818–819

Kaiser-McCaw B, Hecht F (1982) Ataxia telangiectasia: chromosomes and cancer. In: Bridges BA, Harnden DG (eds) Ataxia telangiectasia: a cellular and molecular link between cancer, neuropathology and immune deficiency. Wiley, Chichester, pp 243–257

Kennaugh A, Butterworth S, Hollis R, Baer P, Rabbits TH, Taylor AMR (1986) The chromosome breakpoint at 14q32 in an ataxia-telangiectasia t(14;14) T cell clone is different from the 14q32 breakpoint in Burkitt's and inversion T cell lymphoma. Hum Genet (in press)

Knudson AG (1971) Mutation and cancer: statistical study of retinoblastoma. Proc Natl Acad Sci USA 68:820–823

Krontiris TG, DiMartino NA, Colb M, Parkinson DR (1985) Unique allelic restriction fragments of the human Ha-ras locus in leukocyte and tumour DNAs of cancer patients. Nature 313:369–374

Kunkel LM (1986) Analysis of deletions in DNA from patients with Becker and Duchenne muscular dystrophy. Nature 322:73–77

Lalande M, Dryja TP, Schreck J, Shipley J, Flint A, Latt SA (1984) Isolation of chromosome 13 specific DNA sequences cloned from flow sorted chromosomes and potentially linked to the retinoblastoma locus. Cancer Genet Cytogenet 13:283–296

Lynch HT, Frichot BC, Lynch JF (1977a) Cancer control in xeroderma pigmentosum. Arch Dermatol 113:193–195

Lynch HT, Lynch J, Lynch P (1977b) Management and control of familial cancer. In: Mulvihill JJ, Miller RW, Fraumeni JF (eds) Genetics of human cancer. Raven, New York

Lynch HT, Kimberling WJ, Biscone KA, Lynch JF, Wagner CA, Brennan K, Malliard JA, Johnson PS, Soori JS, McKenna PJ (1986) Familial heterogeneity of colon cancer risk. Cancer 57:2089–2096

Mann JR, Corkery JJ, Fisher HJW, Cameron AH, Mayerova A, Wolf U, Kennaugh AA, Woolley V (1983) The X-linked recessive form of XY gonadal dysgenesis with a high incidence of gonadal germ cell tumours: clinical and genetic studies. J Med Genet 20:264–270

McConnell RB (1966) The genetics of gastrointestinal disorders. Oxford University Press, London

McKusick VA (1983) Mendelian inheritance in man, 6th edn. John Hopkins, Baltimore

Miller RW (1970) Neoplasia and Down's syndrome. Ann NY Acad Sci 171:637–644

Mulvihill JJ (1981) Cancer control through genetics. In: Arrighi FE, Rao PN, Stubblefield E (eds) Genes, chromosomes and neoplasia. Raven, New York

Mulvihill J, Wade WM, Miller RW (1975) Letter: gonadoblastoma in dysgenetic gonads with a Y chromosome. Lancet 1:863

Ponder BAJ (1984) Role of genetics and familial factors. In: Stoll BA (ed) Risk factors and multiple cancer. Wiley, Chichester, pp 177–204

Ramsay CA, Coltart TM, Blunt S, Pawsey SA (1974) Prenatal diagnosis of xeroderma pigmentosum, report of the first successful case. Lancet 2:1109

Ray JH, German J (1981) In: The chromosome changes in Bloom's syndrome, ataxia-telangiectasia, and Fanconi's anaemia. Raven, New York, pp 351–378

Riccardi VM, Hittner HM, Francke U, Yunis JJ, Ledbetter D, Borges W (1980) The aniridia-Wilm's tumour association; the critical role of chromosome band 11p13. Cancer Genet Cytogenet 2:131

Sjoqvist F (1985) Interindividual differences in drug responses: an overview. In: Rowland M, Steiner LB, Steiner JL (eds) Variability in drug therapy: description, estimation and control. Raven, New York

Spector BD, Filipovich AH, Perry GS, Kersey JH (1982) Epidemiology of cancer in ataxia-telangiectasia. In: Bridges BA, Harnden DG (eds) Ataxia-telangiectasia – a cellular and molecular link between cancer, neuropathology and immune deficiency. Wiley, Chichester, pp 103–138

Taub R, Kirsch I, Morton C, Lenoir G, Swan D, Tronick S, Aaronson S, Leder P (1983) Translocation of the *c-myc* gene into the immunoglobulin heavy chain locus in human Burkitt's lymphoma and murine plasmacytoma cells. Proc Nat Acad Sci USA 79:7837–7841

Thein SL, Oscier DG, Flint J, Wainscoat JS (1986) Ha-ras hypervariable alleles in myelodysplasia. Nature 321:84–85

Thorgeirsson SS, Nebert DW (1977) The AL locus and the metabolism of chemical carcinogens and other foreign compounds. Adv Cancer Res 25:149–194

Waterhouse J, Muir C, Correa P, Powell J, Davies W (1976) Cancer incidence in five continents. IARC scientific publication 5. International Agency for Research on Cancer, Lyon

The Role of Epidemiology in the Detection and Reduction of Cancer Risks

R. Doll

Introduction

Epidemiology, that is the study of the variation in the incidence of disease under the conditions of life experienced by different groups of people, has been one of the most productive sources of information about the causes of cancer in man. It has demonstrated that all cancers that are at all common anywhere in the world vary in incidence with place, time, or social group (and often with all three) in such a way that, with few exceptions, very little of the variation can be attributed to group differences in genetic susceptibility, however important such differences may be in distinguishing between the risks to individuals within each group. It has, moreover, demonstrated that these differences are so large that some 80% or 90% of all the cancers that occur annually throughout the world must, in principle, be avoidable.

Sometimes these differences have led directly to the detection of a specific cause, as has happened following the observation of an excess risk associated with a particular occupation, and sometimes they have led to a similar result indirectly by providing clues that have guided more detailed epidemiological or laboratory investigation, as in the discovery of the relationship between tobacco and lung cancer and between the Epstein-Barr (EB) virus and Burkitt's lymphoma. By such means observation of differences in incidence has, in one way or another, played a part in the detection of the majority of the 40-odd causes of human cancer that have already been detected.

We are not, however, concerned here with the past, except in so far as experience of the past can help to guide our work in the future, and I shall review the role of epidemiology only in relation to the development of practical measures for the avoidance of those causes that have already been identified and in the detection of the many others that await discovery. I have referred, it will be noted, to the causes of cancer rather than to cancer risks. I should, therefore, explain that I am not using cause in the philosophers' sense of something that has to be present for an effect to be produced and is, when present, sufficient to ensure that the effect occurs. I am, rather, using it in the sense given it by those concerned with the practice of public health of something that, when present, increases the risk of developing disease and, when removed, leads to the risk being reduced. It is in this second sense that I shall always refer to cause, giving to risk, the definition recommended by a study group of the Royal Society (1983): that is, the probability that a particular adverse event occurs during a stated period of time or results from a particular challenge.

Measures for the Prevention of Cancer Due to Known Causes

Occasionally the cause that has been discovered has been a manmade chemical that could be replaced without great difficulty and its manufacture and use have quickly ceased, as in the case of chlornaphazine, a drug that was used to treat polycythaemia and was soon found to cause cancer of the bladder. More often the cause has also had other effects, some of which have been useful or enjoyable and not easily obtainable in other ways, as with tobacco, alcohol, asbestos, and ionizing radiations, or the cause has been produced inadvertently by activities that are socially important, as with the polycyclic hydrocarbons that are produced by the combustion of fossil fuel. In these circumstances prevention involves social costs that may be substantial and socially controversial and total elimination of the risk may be impracticable. Epidemiological observation continues, therefore, to be needed to see if the measures imposed are having the desired effect. Consider, for example, the measures taken to reduce the risk from smoking, to control exposure to ionizing radiations, and to prevent hepatocellular carcinoma.

Tobacco

Measures imposed to restrict smoking have varied from one country to another and have had different impacts on the amount smoked. Their success or failure, as measured by tobacco sales, poses problems for sociological and economic research. We cannot, however, suppose that any practicable measures will eliminate smoking altogether within the forseeable future and it has to be asked whether, as an interim measure, cigarettes can be manufactured that are less hazardous than the regular cigarettes of the past. Case-control studies, such as that of Lubin et al. (1984) which included nearly 8000 cases of lung cancer in five European countries, suggest that they can be (Table 1) and so does the American Cancer Society's massive cohort study of 1 million Americans (Hammond et al. 1976). The interpretation of these studies is,

Table 1. Relative risk of lung cancer by use of high and low tar brand cigarettes (after Lubin et al. 1984)

Brand of cigarette[a]	Percent of smoking history	Relative risk[b]	
		Men	Women
Low tar	100	1.00	1.00
Low tar	>75	1.2	–
Mixed	–	1.5	5.9
High tar	>75	1.8	4.0
High tar	100	1.7	7.7

[a] Not adjusted for use of filters
[b] Standardized for years of cigarette use, number smoked per day, and years since cessation

Table 2. Change in mortality from lung cancer in men under 50 years of age (England and Wales, 1950–1984)

Age (years)	Mortality per million men per year			Reduction (%)
	1951–1955	1956–1960	1983–1984	
30–34	*38*	37	11	71
35–39	*101*	95	38	62
40–44	253	*256*	114	56
45–49	589	*597*	296	50

however, complicated by confounding the type of cigarette smoked with the reasons for choosing it. As, moreover, there has been very little reduction in the mortality from lung cancer, even in early middle age, in many countries in which the average tar content of cigarette smoke has been substantially reduced, the value of restricting tar levels has been questioned (National Research Council 1982). Cigarette smoke, however, contains both initiating agents as well as promoting agents and no big reduction can yet be expected in countries such as the USA where the average amount smoked continued to increase until 1950 or later. In other countries where the amount smoked by young men had stabilized before World War II, as in Great Britain and Finland, the reduction in the amount of tar delivered per cigarette has been followed by a sharp reduction in the mortality from lung cancer, most marked in those whose smoking histories have been confined to the reduced tar era (Table 2), and which began 15 years before there was any material reduction in the amount smoked (Kiryluk et al. 1986).

Ionizing Radiations

The second set of measures, to limit the extent of exposure to ionizing radiations, has depended mainly on quantitative estimates of what the risks are likely to be. Crucial though laboratory investigation is to avoid the introduction of new carcinogens into the environment, there is as yet no reliable way of extrapolating risks quantitatively from laboratory animals to man, and, if carcinogens have to be used, we can estimate the risk associated with a given level of exposure only by direct observation or by extrapolation from the risk observed at other levels.

Until recently the only quantitative data available for the effects of ionizing radiations were obtained from observation of people exposed acutely to large doses of low linear energy transfer (LET) radiation either from the atomic bomb explosions in Japan (Darby et al. 1985b) or from the experience of patients treated by radiotherapy, in particular the experience of 14000 patients treated for ankylosing spondylitis in the UK between 1935 and 1954 (Court-Brown and Doll 1965; Darby et al. 1987). Fortunately, all sets of data give broadly similar results, once allowance is made for the fact that the very high doses received locally from radiotherapy kill cells as well as causing mutations in them, and all the national and international committees that have used these data to estimate the effects of small doses have concluded that 10 mSv (1 rem) would cause between 80 and 300 cancer deaths in every 1 million exposed persons, with the International Commission for Radiation Protection (1977) giving a figure of 125 deaths, which is somewhat nearer the lower than the upper end of the range.

The value of these estimates for control purposes depends on the validity of two assumptions: (a) that high doses received in a matter of seconds or less have much the same carcinogenic effect as the same doses spread out over periods of days, months, or years, and (b) that the relative biological efficiency in man of low LET radiation (X and gamma rays and beta particles) and of high LET radiation (neutrons and alpha particles) are known adequately from animal experiments. These assumptions are, unfortunately, more a matter of faith than of established fact and it is important to observe what actually happens in industrial practice. Large numbers of subjects will have to be observed for very long periods before we can be sure of the results, but the data now available for the workers at the Hanford plant in the USA, where plutonium has been processed, and for the employees of the Atomic Energy Authority in the UK (Tolley et al. 1983; Beral et al. 1985) which together relate to more than 50000 men, most of whom have been observed for over 20 years, provide in combination estimates of risk that lie between no effect at all and 10 times that predicted by the International Commission. It is encouraging, however, to note that the best estimates obtained from this industrial experience for both leukaemia and for all fatal cancers are just about 1½ times as great as those derived from the experience of the bomb survivors and the patients given radiotherapy (Darby et al. 1985a). These findings justify, at least for the time being, the continued use of a figure very close to the internationally accepted prediction for control purposes and suggest that background radiation in the UK, now considered to be about 1.8 mSv per person per year when account is taken of the radon that accumulates in underventilated houses, contributes to approximately 1.6% of all fatal cancers in the country if, as I prefer, the ICRP estimate is doubled.

Continued observation is, however, essential, as a few observations have been made that do not fit the pattern, notably the excess of leukaemia in the participants of one series of nuclear test explosions in the USA (Robinette et al. 1985) and the increased incidence of childhood leukaemia in the vicinity of two British nuclear reactors (Black 1984; Heasman et al. 1985). Until these observations are explained the subject cannot be regarded as closed.

Hepatitis B Virus

My third example of the continued need for epidemiological observation in the practical application of current knowledge is provided by the programmes now planned or actually initiated for the prevention of hepatocellular carcinoma by immunization. The results of the cohort study that Beasley et al. (1981) are conducting in Taiwan, in conjunction with results of many case-control studies, leave no serious doubt that the hepatitis B virus is a cause of the majority of cases of hepatocellular carcinoma throughout the world and that the disease is virtually limited to carriers of the virus; but the virus has not been shown to cause cancer in primates and does not satisfy the criteria that Henle (1971) proposed for concluding that a virus is the cause of human cancer – as applied in relation to the EB virus and Burkitt's lymphoma and cancer of the nasopharynx. We should, therefore, check that an immunization programme actually achieves the desired result. The evidence to inculpate the carrier state is too strong for a controlled trial with random allocation to be ethical given that sufficient supplies of vaccine are available, now that we know that the carrier state can be effectively prevented by immunization at or soon after birth (Beasley et al. 1983) and the International Agency for Research on Cancer (1985) is, therefore, seeking to achieve a convincing result in its trial of immunization in the Gambia by a programme that will move progressively from one area to another and cover the whole country in 4 years. Knowledge of the age and place of birth of an individual should then make it possible to tell, in 20–30 years' time, whether he was immunized or not. The same method will, I understand, also be used in China when, in 1990, sufficient supplies of vaccine are expected to become available at trivial cost, as a result of the genetic engineering that enables large amounts of a viral antigen to be produced in yeast.

Hepatocellular carcinoma begins to become common at a relatively early age in tropical countries, but even so it must be the best part of 25 years before any clear result is obtained and it does not seem justifiable to wait so long before taking any other action, if any other action might be expected to reduce the risk of the disease more quickly. One such action would be to reduce the amount of aflatoxin in the diet by better storage (or controlled importation) of staple oil-bearing foods, as the close geographical correlation between the incidence of hepatocellular carcinoma and the amount of aflatoxin in the diet suggests that aflatoxin also needs to be present before much disease occurs (van Rensburg et al. 1985; Yeh et al. 1983). It is, therefore, to be hoped that efforts to reduce the aflatoxin content of the diet will also be made in all countries where liver cancer is common and that the effect will be monitored by regular measurement of the metabolites of aflatoxin in the urine of representative samples of the population.

Detection of New Causes of Cancer

The causes of cancer that are known and are, in one way or another, capable of avoidance account for about one-third of all the cancers that now occur annually throughout the world and will account for over 40% if, as seems extremely likely, melanomas prove to be mostly due to exposure of the untanned skin to ultraviolet light and cervical cancer to infection with some specific types of the human papilloma virus. Melanomas have increased in incidence steadily for many years in all fair-skinned populations, but even so they are still relatively uncommon. Cervical cancer, by contrast, is probably the second most common cancer in women throughout the world and the seventh most common in both sexes combined. Even with these additions to the list of preventable cancers, there will, however, still remain three of the most common cancers (that is cancers of the stomach, breast, and large bowel) and many less common ones whose causes are largely unknown despite the existence of many tantalizing clues.

In this situation epidemiology can continue to play an important role, partly by the continued application of old techniques, but perhaps most importantly by their further development in closer conjunction with laboratory scientists.

Monitoring Differences in Cancer Incidence

It is unlikely that much more will be learned from geographical differences in incidence, except perhaps from the variation that is now realized to occur in China. A national survey of cancer mortality for the years 1973–1975 revealed substantial differences in the pattern of mortality between 30 provinces and large towns, with the biggest differences being recorded for those cancers that are also very variable in the rest of the world and relatively small differences being recorded for other cancers such as leukaemia and cancers of the breast and brain which are relatively constant elsewhere (Table 3). Much greater differences were observed between smaller areas, but although some of these are certainly real, such as the hundred-fold differences recorded in the mortality from cancers of the oesophagus and nasopharynx, much of this variation is likely to be due to random variation and to differences in the accuracy of certification of death. The opportunity provided by these observations has been seized in a most imaginative manner by Chen, Campbell, Peto, and Li (personal communication) who have organized a survey of representative samples of 50 men and 50 women in each of 65 counties chosen to provide some of the biggest contrasts between the mortality rates for 20 types of cancer. In this survey questions have been asked about various aspects of personal behaviour and samples of blood, urine, and food have been collected. These samples have been distributed to 10 specialist laboratories in four countries and it will soon be possible to compare cancer

Table 3. Variation in cancer mortality: 30 parts of China (Editorial Committee for the Atlas of Cancer Mortality 1979)

Type of cancer	Maximum annual death rate per 100000		Ratio of maximum to minimum rates	
	Males	Females	Males	Females
Oesophagus	70.9	36.7	33	33
Nasopharynx	12.5	5.0	22	10
Bladder	3.7	1.1	8	16
Lung	42.2	14.3	12	9
Stomach	81.2	42.2	8	9
Lymphoma	2.7	1.2	12	3
Cervix	–	29.4	–	7
Liver	39.1	15.0	5	4
Colon and rectum	11.4	9.3	4	5
Leukaemia	4.4	3.5	4	5
Breast	–	6.0	–	4
Brain	2.6	2.2	3	3

mortality rates with some 200-odd variables including more than 150 biological measurements of current interest.

It is, of course, important to continue monitoring the incidence of cancer through the mechanism of cancer registries, particularly now that treatment is becoming more effective and at last beginning to influence the trends in mortality. I doubt, however, that we can expect to obtain early warning of any new hazard in this way very often as it is difficult to be sure about the meaning of small changes in the incidence of common cancers, and rare cancers such as pleural mesothelioma and hepatic angiosarcoma, are seldom recorded separately until after a new cause has been detected. Cancer registration data are, I suspect, likely to be more useful in monitoring the effect of measures introduced for the control of cancer and in providing research workers with access to information about individual cases. There is, however, no knowing when cancer is going to spring a new surprise on us, like the increase in cervical cancer in young women that has occurred in cohorts that reached sexual maturity around 1960 and which appears so starkly in the national mortality rates for England and Wales (Doll 1985).

Epidemiological observation is certainly not the method of choice for detecting new chemical hazards, which should be avoided by laboratory investigation of new agents before they are introduced. Variation in the susceptibility of animal species and the possibility that noncarcinogenic chemicals may interact in an unexpected way in an industrial process or in vivo means, however, that some new causes of cancer are always liable to escape the net and we ought to monitor the incidence of cancer in all major industries that handle new materials and in patients exposed to new drugs, as well as in society as a whole.

Analytical Epidemiology

The most important role for epidemiology – and the most difficult to predict – remains the investigation of the causes of those common cancers whose causes are still unknown. These, I suspect, are most likely to be dietary and metabolic, hormonal, and viral, and none of them is easy to investigate by epidemiological means alone.

A clue to a possible viral cause may be provided by the occurrence of case-clusters like those that were reported for Burkitt's lymphoma. It has occasionally been obtained for acute lymphoblastic leukaemia of childhood (Till et al. 1967), but I doubt that we can expect to find it for any other precise type of cancer, unless we do for some other types of acute leukaemia or lymphoma. I doubt too that we can obtain for any other cancer clear indirect evidence of infectivity like that obtained when cervical cancer was shown to relate to the number of sexual partners of the affected woman's partner. All epidemiology can hope to do in this field is, I suspect, to demonstrate differences in incidence in cohort studies when laboratory investigation has provided evidence of specific viral infection.

Epidemiology should, however, be more helpful in the other fields if it can be combined more intimately with laboratory investigation. There must, for example, be a lot more that can be learned from study of the blood levels of hormones in groups of women with different expectations of developing breast cancer, taking into account not only their age, but also the length of their menstrual cycle and the day of the cycle when the measurement was made and similar investigations during pregnancy may, as Depue et al. (1983) suggest, throw light on the origin of testicular cancer in young men. For this purpose, as for the investigation of dietary factors, we should, I believe, provide for the collection and maintenance of large banks of biological samples similar to but more extensive than the one collected by Chen et al. (personal communication) in China, and including samples of cells from buccal and cervical smears and from blood. Preliminary findings from simple serum banks have already effectively eliminated serum levels of retinol and cholesterol as significant markers of cancer risk in developed countries, but have left open the possibility of protective effects of beta carotene, selenium, and vitamin E and have drawn attention to the possible importance of derivatives of male sex hormones in relation to cancer of the breast.

Rather than generalize further, I shall conclude by referring to the potential for combined epidemiological and laboratory research into the possible role of nitrates and nitrites in the aetiology of oesophageal and gastric cancer. The question is important partly because these two types of cancer are so common – oesophageal cancer being the most common type of lethal cancer in several parts of Africa and Asia and gastric cancer being the second most common in the world as a whole – and partly because the nitrate content of water is tending to rise and the measures required to restrict it, even to the new levels now laid down by the EEC, will cost many millions of pounds.

That nitrates as well as nitrites may lead to the production of nitrosamines in vivo is clear; but the evidence relating either to the development of cancer in man is conflicting. A close correlation, for example, is found between gastric cancer and dietary nitrate in different countries (Hartman 1983), while in Britain no correlation is found between gastric cancer and nitrates in water supplies (Beresford 1985) nor in the saliva of representative samples of the local population (Forman et al. 1985) and no excess of gastric cancer is found in men employed in the manufacture of nitrate fertilizers (Al-Dabbagh et al. 1986). None of these observations are, however, sufficiently direct to be decisive and we need also to have measures of the ability of samples of each population to form nitrosamines in vivo when exposed to equal amounts of the nitrate and nitrite substrates. One way in which such a measure can be obtained is by giving measured amounts of proline and seeing how much is excreted as nitrosoproline in the urine (Oshima and Bartsch 1981). There are, of course, other ways in which the ability to form nitrosamines can be measured, and I have cited the use of the nitrosoproline test only as an example of the sort of way in which epidemiology must, I think, develop if it is to make many more major contributions to the detection of new causes of the common cancers of still unknown aetiology.

Conclusion

In this brief review, I have summarized the past contributions of epidemiology in two paragraphs and have tried, in the rest, to look forward to the ways in which it may contribute in the future. Others interested in the field might well paint a different picture, but we would all agree that the contribution that epidemiology is still capable of making is substantial. It is important, however, not to expect more of it than it can provide. Epidemiology cannot tell us that any particular material is safe in the absolute sense and it is much more likely than laboratory science to overlook small effects of the many thousand chemicals that are used in modern society. By starting, however, from the thousands of cases of cancer that actually occur each year, it is much less likely to overlook the large determinants of risks and trends and provides the only conclusive evidence that our policies for the avoidance of cancer are soundly based.

References

Al-Dabbagh S, Forman D, Bryson D, Stratton I, Doll R (1986) Mortality of nitrate fertiliser workers. Br J Indust Med 43:507–519

Beasley RP, Hwang LY, Lin CC, Chien SC (1981) Hepatocellular carcinoma and Hepatitus B virus: a prospective study of 22,707 women in Taiwan. Lancet 2:1129–1133

Beasley RP, Hwang LY, Lee GCY, Lan CC, Roan CH, Huang F, Chen CL (1983) Prevention of perinatally transmitted Hepatitis B virus infections with Hepatitis B immune globulin and Hepatitis B vaccine. Lancet 2:1099–1102

Beral V, Inskip H, Fraser P, Booth M, Coleman D, Rose G (1985) Mortality of employees of the United Kingdom Atomic Energy Authority, 1946–1979. Br Med J 291:440–447

Beresford SAA (1985) Is nitrate in the drinking water associated with the risk of cancer of the urban U.K.? Int J Epidemiol 14:57–63

Black D (ed) (1984) Investigation of the possible increased incidence of cancer in Cumbria. Her Majesty's Stationery Office, London

Court-Brown WM, Doll R (1965) Mortality from cancer and other causes after radiotherapy for ankylosing spondylitis. Br Med J 2:1327–1332

Darby SC, Doll R, Pike MC (1985a) Mortality of employees of the United Kingdom Atomic Energy Authority, 1946–1979. Br Med J 291:672

Darby SC, Nakashima E, Kato H (1985b) A parallel analysis of cancer mortality among atomic bomb survivors and patients with ankylosing spondylitis given X-ray therapy. JNCI 75:1–21

Darby SC, Doll R, Gill SK, Smith PG (1987) Mortality after a single treatment course with X-rays in patients treated for ankylosing spondylitis. Br J Cancer

Depue RH (1984) Maternal and gestational factors affecting the risk of cryptorchidism and inguinal hernia. Int J Epidemiol 13:311–318

Depue RH, Pike MC, Henderson BE (1983) Estrogen exposure during gestation and risk of testicular cancer. JNCI 71:1151–1155

Doll R (1985) Invasive cervical cancer and combined oral contraceptives. Br Med J 290:1210

Editorial Committee for the Atlas of Cancer Mortality (1979) Atlas of cancer mortality in the People's Republic of China. China Map Press, Shanghai

Forman D, Al-Dabbagh S, Doll R (1985) Nitrates, nitrites and gastric cancer in Great Britain. Nature 313:620–625

Hammond C, Garfinkel L, Seidman H, Lew EA (1976) Tar and nicotine content of cigarette smoke in relation to death rates. Environ Res 12:263–274

Hartman PE (1983) Nitrates/nitrites and gastric cancer. Environ Mutagen 5:111–121

Heasman MA, Kemp IW, Urquhart JD, Black R (1986) Childhood leukaemia in Northern Scotland. Lancet 1:266

Henle W (1971) Evidence for a relation of the Epstein-Barr virus to Burkitt's lymphoma and nasopharyngeal carcinoma. In: Recent Advances in Human Tumor Virology and Immunology (Proceedings of the 1st International Symposium of the Princess Takamatsu Cancer Research Fund), Tokyo University Press, Tokyo, pp 361–367

International Agency for Research on Cancer (1985) Annual report. International Agency for Research on Cancer, Lyon

International Commission on Radiological Protection (1977) Recommendations of the international commission on radiological protection. Pergamon, Oxford

Kiryluk S, Wald N, Darby SC, Doll R, Peto R (eds) (1986) UK Smoking statistics. Oxford University Press, Oxford (in press)
Lubin JH, Blot WJ, Berrino F, Flamant R, Gillis CRK, Kunze M, Schmahl D, Visco G (1984) Patterns of lung cancer according to type of cigarette smoked. Int J Cancer 33:569–576
National Research Council (1982) Reduced tar and nicotine cigarettes. National Research Council, National Academy Press, Washington, DC
Oshima H, Bartsch H (1981) Quantitative estimates of endogenous nitrosation in humans by monitoring N-nitrosoproline excretion in the urine. Cancer Res 41:3658–3662
Robinette CD, Jablon S, Preston TL (1985) Mortality of nuclear weapons test participants. National Research Council, National Academy Press, Washington, DC
Till MM, Hardisty RM, Pike MC, Doll R (1967) Childhood leukaemia in Greater London: a search for evidence of clustering. Br Med J 2:755–758
Tolley KD, Marks S, Buchanan JA, Gilberts ES (1983) A further update of the analysis of mortality of workers in a nuclear facility. Radiat Res 95:211–213
van Rensburg SJ, Cook-Mozaffari P, van Schalkwyk DJ, van der Watt JJ, Vincent TJ, Purchase IF (1985) Hepatocellular carcinoma and dietary aflatoxin in Mozambique and Transkei. Br J Cancer 51:713–726
Yeh FS, Yan RC, Mor CC, Liu YK, Yang KC (1983) Research on aetiological factors of hepatocellular carcinoma in Guangsci, China. In: Proceedings of the 13th international cancer congress, Seattle, p 340

Summary of Discussion: Session 1

L. Arab-Kohlmeier

In recognition of the increased risk of cancer in individuals homozygotic for certain diseases, the discussion centered around whether or not heterozygote recessive syndromes are also associated with an increased cancer risk. Ataxia-telangiectasia and xeroderma pigmentosum, according to Professor Harnden, are associated with an increased cancer risk in heterozygotes at a young age, but the case in other diseases is not clear. It was pointed out that if heterozygotes do have an increased risk, this may explain a considerable amount of the variability in cancer susceptibility of the population. For example ataxia-telangiectasia is known to be nonhomogeneously distributed.

If it were homogeneous, and heterozygotes were endangered, approximately 1% of the population would be at risk. In contrast, it is estimated that 2%–3% of the population is at risk because of the nonhomogeneous background of this disorder.

Then the question was posed whether information had been obtained through the birth records of noble families about their possibly increased cancer risk. Studies on familial cancer in noble families had not been heard of.

The question of whether Burkitt's cell informers in ataxia-telangiectasia patients show a rearrangement of the immunoglobulin genes was asked. As most of the tests on these patients were conducted prior to the availability of the methodology for examining rearrangement of genes, no information on this topic is currently available.

Differences in susceptibility of different animal strains to liver cancer were discussed. The extent to which these genetic differences in experimental systems have contributed to the understanding of the genetics of cancer was queried. In response it was noted that the animal strains were bred specifically for their susceptibility, and furthermore, variability in the population was eliminated; consequently, studies of genetics using these animals are not widely applicable.

Sir Richard Doll was asked why his presentation on the role of epidemiology in detecting and preventing cancer did not include reference to the potential of applied epidemiology, and whether or not he believed this belonged within the field of epidemiology. He responded that he does believe it to be a part of epidemiology and did not include it because he felt confident it would be discussed in the sessions on tobacco smoking and cancer.

Discussion of the two documented clusters of leukemia around nuclear plant sites in England took place. The belief was expressed by Sir Richard Doll that these are not radiation linked, based on the nondetectable increase of leukemia after comparable or higher levels of radioactive fallout of the 1950s. Furthermore, he believes that the evidence is becoming increasingly convincing that leukemia is of a viral origin and these isolated communities are demonstrating epidemics of the same.

SESSION 2

Chemical Carcinogens: Risk Assessment

Chairman: D. Neubert

Assessment of Cancer Risk from Chemicals

D. HENSCHLER

Introduction

Induction of cancer by exposure to chemicals was disclosed 127 years before the first report of cancer from X-rays (Frieben 1902), and 136 years before the unequivocal establishment of viruses as cancer-causing agents (Rous 1911). Percival Pott (1775) is generally credited with having described the first chemically induced occupational cancer, in chimney sweepers after long-term exposure to soot, followed later on by reports of coal tar being causally related to skin cancer (Volkmann 1875). Another pioneer contribution was by Rehn in 1895 who described bladder cancer in dye-stuff workers for the first time. He ascribed these cancers to aniline but, as we now know, they were induced by β-naphthylamine and benzidine.

Occupational Cancer: No Special Case

It is not by chance that chemical carcinogenesis continued to be greatly influenced for quite a while by observations in occupational medicine of cancer caused by exposure to chemicals. Nickel, chromate, arsenic, 4-amino-biphenyl, asbestos, and benzene are additional examples which entered the scientific literature rather slowly – long before systematic animal experiments were initiated. Those who are engaged today in the business of carcinogenicity testing of chemicals in experimental animals, adding compound after compound to the ever-increasing list of proven animal carcinogens, only too easily forget that the main criteria of chemically induced cancer, namely organ specificity, latency period, multiplicity of tumor formation, and dependence on dose were established by these early observers of occupational tumors, sometimes based on just a few case studies.

Another interesting feature becomes obvious when one looks at these early reports by occupational physicians. There is no awareness of cancer being a specific issue in the wide spectrum of diseases. The irreversibility of carcinogenic lesions, the poor curability of occupationally induced cancers were not paid special attention. Indeed, cancer incidences in industry, however high in a specific location they might have been, constituted only a small fraction of the overall rate of occupational diseases and accidents. Also, the pioneers in this field held the belief that cancer could be prevented, or at least considerably reduced by interruption of exposure or intermittent exposure-free periods.

Alertness Arising from New Observations

A change of this conventional attitude was only induced by a series of grave experiences in the 1960s and 1970s:

1. Hemangiosarcomas occurring in workers exposed to vinyl chloride as long as 4 decades after the introduction of the compound as a bulk chemical (Creech and Johnson 1974)
2. Mesotheliomas and bronchial cancer at high rates after asbestos exposure, again with the extremely long latency period of 4 decades and more (Wagner et al. 1960)
3. Bronchial carcinomas at an extremely high rate in small groups of workers who had been exposed, sometimes for very short periods of time only, to bis(-chloromethyl) ether (Thiess et al. 1973).

From then on, chemically induced occupational cancer was recognized as a disease of special dimension. This change of mind was accompanied and certainly influenced in part by the introduction of systematic carcinogenicity testing with experimental animals. Although some forerunners demonstrating carcinogenic effects of chemicals or of complex mixtures date back to the beginning of the century (Yamagiwa and Ichikawa 1911), it was again not until the 1960s that systematic approaches were established which exceeded experimental efforts in the context of scientific interest, such as the work of Druckrey and his group to whom special credit should be given. In the course of just a few years, to be dated around 1965, large programs for animal carcinogenicity testing brought about a formalization of the procedures and led to the introduction of fixed protocols. As a result of these activities which were mostly carried out in the USA and a few other highly industrialized countries, the number of identified animal carcinogens grew rapidly but only occasionally was a new member chemical added to the list of those compounds found to produce cancer in humans.

Classification Systems

Despite rapid, or better, dramatic development, classification systems have kept to the traditional pattern of distinguishing between human carcinogens, given first place, and animal carcinogens in the second. I wish to introduce two existing systems of classifying carcinogens which may present, above the common basis of the hierarchy human over animal, differences in the validation of methods and in the evaluation of results: the IARC system – see the IARC monograph series, vol. 1 (1972) to vol. 38 (1986) – and the German System – as established by the DFG Commission for the Investigation of Health Hazards of Chemical Compounds in the Work Area (DFG 1958–1986).

The IARC system has been oscillating over the years, and repeatedly amplified or corrected according to the newest information or insights by work groups with an ever-changing composition. It distinguishes clearly between assessment of existing data and evaluation of risk to humans. The sources of information are differentiated as to

1. Human data (case reports, descriptive and analytical epidemiology)
2. Experimental animal data (species and strains, routes of administration, tumor incidence for new sites and types, as well as increase of rate and decrease of time of appearance of spontaneous tumors)
3. Short-term tests (number of tests applied, number of positive vs negative results, levels of genetic damage)

The assessment makes a classification for each of these sources according to: sufficient evidence, limited evidence, inadequate evidence, no evidence (no data available).

The evaluation of carcinogenic risk to humans is then subdivided into four groups:

Group 1: Carcinogenic to humans (sufficient evidence from human studies)
Group 2A: Probably carcinogenic to humans (limited evidence from human studies, mostly sufficient evidence from animal studies)
Group 2B: Less probably carcinogenic to humans (inadequate human data, sufficient evidence from animal studies)
Group 3: Cannot be classified (inadequate evidence in humans, animals and short-term tests)

This system has advantages and disadvantages. A positive element may be seen in the consensus that has been achieved within an international group of experts on the assessment of data from different sources. This will lead, however, also to inconsistencies in judgment from volume to volume produced because the recruitment of experts varies widely. This manifests itself particularly in a rather inconstant attribution of compounds to Groups 2A and 2B, groups which in fact lack a clear-cut definition. What should a national authority conclude from the classification of "less probability of being carcinogenic to humans" for regulatory purposes? This obvious weakness of the system clearly is due to the overemphasis put on formal aspects of data evaluation of long-term animal carcinogenicity studies, such as tumor classification, statistical treatment of results, survival time, etc. In general, the IARC system refuses to take into account mechanistic considerations of chemical carcinogenesis. The four evaluation groups are, as they stand, not suitable for regulatory purposes. In fact, one finds quite a number of contradictory decisions by different national governmental agencies on a given compound.

The German system tries to overcome some of these difficulties in that it does not subdivide the evidence of risk to humans into three groups. The classification system which was introduced in its present form in 1976 provides three categories:

IIIA(1): Working materials capable of inducing malignant tumors as shown by experience with humans
IIIA(2): Compounds which in the Commission's opinion have proven so far to be unmistakably carcinogenic in animal experimentation only; namely, under conditions which are comparable to those for possible exposure of a human being at the workplace, or from which such comparability can be deduced
IIIB: Compounds which are justifiably suspected of having carcinogenic potential and which urgently need further investigation

Categories IIIA(1) and IIIA(2) are not differentiated for regulatory purposes, which is in line with the internationally established principle that unequivocally positive findings in animal experiments should be regarded as if they pose a carcinogenic hazard for humans. In other words, the distinction between human and animal carcinogens is irrelevant for risk estimation and cancer prevention. Category IIIB is not regulated as (proven) carcinogens, but it constitutes a warning to individuals at exposure in the work area as well as to employers and authorities, and it enjoins a search for better alternatives as well as further research to clarify the situation, which means either substantiation or rejection of the suspicion raised.

Pros and Cons of the Two Classification Systems

The German system differs in several respects from the IARC pattern in that: (a) it does not accept animal data obtained from experiments with improper dose regimens and routes of administration; (b) there is no formalization with regard to species, strain, and number of experiments performed; (c) it takes into account mechanistic considerations such as chemical analogy, bioactivation mechanisms, and reactivity of ultimate carcinogens; and (d) it allows for rapid inclusion of the results of scientific progress.

In fact, the German list of occupational carcinogens contains more compounds than the IARC list, in part due to the more flexible decision-making criteria, but mostly because it is possible to act and react more quickly to new information on the national level than the international.

Insufficiencies of Classification Policies

One disadvantage is common to both systems, as is the case with all systems exercised worldwide. This becomes obvious if one looks at the dynamics of the expansion of the existing groups or categories. There has been hardly any addition to the group of proven human carcinogens over the past 1–2 decades, whereas the list of proven animal carcinogens is ever-increasing in an exponential manner and even more so is the list of suspected carcinogens. At present, the German MAK List nominates approximately 150 proven or suspected carcinogens which constitutes one third of all listed occupational chemicals. If this tendency of increase continues in the years to come, and there is no indication of a reduction or steady state, we will soon have more carcinogens than noncarcinogens.

There are two major reasons for this phenomenon. The first is the high testing activity and capacity, to a great extent established and sponsored in the United States in the form of the NCI/NTP Program which continuously provides relevant data to satisfy the zeal of those who are charged with assessment and evaluation of risk. The second results from the inflexibility of the existing policies practised in classifying carcinogens. This policy implies that there are no thresholds for carcinogens, and hence the only way of preventing or reducing risk is to avoid exposure, or to keep it as low as possible. The real dilemma must be seen in our inability to quantify carcinogenic risks. At present, we do not have scientifically valid instruments to extrapolate quantitatively from animals to humans. We do not even fulfill the minimum requirement for quantification of carcinogenic potency in animals: dose-response relationships. Instead, the protocol, which is applied in the majority of long-term animal carcinogenicity testings, is the use of only two exposure groups: one with the so-called "maximum tolerated dose" (MTD), and a second one with half of it (MTD/2). This protocol only renders information as to a carcinogenic potential (hazard). It does not allow for establishing the slope of a dose-response curve, which is the second pillar of quantification, or for the determination of carcinogenic potency (risk, or probability of cancer incidence in an individual as well as in a population).

Hazard Assessment Vs Risk Evaluation

How then could the generation of quantitative risk data be achieved? The most reliable way is analytical epidemiology. Unfortunately, however, we know of only a few examples where epidemiology has been in a position to establish dose-response relationships which allow for predicting an individual's or a population's risk of developing a certain type of cancer. Examples are tumors from tobacco smoking, hepatic tumors from aflatoxin B_1 intake, and (although with much less precision) leukemia development from occupational exposure to benzene, or bladder tumors after exposure to some aromatic amines. I am afraid that not many more such examples will become available in the foreseeable future, due to the improving strategies of protection and prevention, particularly in occupational premises, which will result in decreasing rates of cancer of this origin. Epidemiology has additional limitations. One of these is being realized right now in the attempt to verify a carcinogenic risk in nonsmokers from passive smoking: although the availability of exposed populations is practically unlimited, the effect to be expected is very low, the tumor to be formed occurs at rather high spontaneous or otherwise induced rate. And much more important for the present and future situation: epidemiology can only go to work after exposure to endangering chemicals has taken place, and results can only be expected after a considerable latency period which in the case of very low doses and cancer incidence rates extends to 2–3 decades or more. This means that with newly introduced chemicals one has to accept a carcinogenic load of unknown dimension before epidemiology can be expected to work successfully.

Therefore, with new chemicals, as well as with many old ones which have not awakened this specific interest so far, we have to look for alternatives. One approach which is practised in some countries is an attempt to extrapolate from animal carcinogenicity data to a preset level of human risk (in terms of tumor incidence) using mathematical models. A variety of models has been proposed all of which have to make a multitude of assumptions because of the unknown shape of the real dose-response curve in the very low-dose range. All of these assumptions lack any biological background. Therefore, the procedures just represent mathematical exercises which cannot take into account, e.g., species differences and so they are charged with a variety of errors the magnitude of which cannot be calculated. These models may satisfy regulators who only too often overemphasize figures and neglect biological facts and who act under political pressure to do something for an improvement of a given situation, rather than to wait for an improvement of the scientific basis.

New Strategies for Risk Extrapolation Needed

The best way towards a more reliable extrapolation of risk from animals to man is to look intensively into the reasons for interspecies differences in the susceptibility to carcinogenic stimuli. This means the study of pharmacokinetics and metabolism of carcinogens, the mechanisms of their interactions with the genetic material at any available level, the fate of primary carcinogenic lesions with time, and the correlation of these with the final tumor formation – all with the aim of interspecies comparisons, man to be included wherever possible. This means that the present type of "bioassay" studies is to be improved, or better say substituted by experiments which take into account these mechanistic elements *before* the start of the life-time study, particularly with regard to selecting out that species which comes closest to humans. One important new technique may bring us a decisive step forward in these efforts towards a more rational and more reliable prediction of risk: biomonitoring of exposure to carcinogens by measuring chemical, biochemical, and biological end-points such as protein- and DNA-adduct formation, cytogenetic changes and even preneoplastic lesions. The closer these end-points in the multistep process of carcinogenesis are to the final tumor manifestation, the more reliable the prediction of risk will be. This means the incorporation of more biology and more science into the existing carcinogenicity testing procedures which up to now are dominated by descriptive morphological and statistical methods. The time seems to be ripe for changes in the protocols and progress is urgently needed in face of the permanent challenge of toxicologists and carcinologists by the dramatic innovation rate of chemists in industry and elsewhere who confront us with an ever-increasing number of new chemicals with sometimes impressively increased biological reactivity and health-impairing potential.

References

Creech JL, Johnson MN (1974) Angiosarcoma of liver in the manufacture of polyvinyl chloride. J Occup Med 16:150

Deutsche Forschungsgemeinschaft (DFG) Commission for the Investigation of Health Hazards of Chemical Compounds in the Work Area (1958–1986) Annual list of maximum concentrations at the workplace. VCH, Weinheim

Frieben H (1902) Ärztlicher Verein Hamburg, meeting of 21 October 1902. Münch Med Wochenschr 49:1820

Pott P (1775) Chirurgical observations and the mortification of the toes and the feet. Hawkes and Collins, London

Rehn L (1895) Blasengeschwülste bei Fuchsinarbeitern. Arch Klin Chir 50:588

Rous P (1911) Transmission of a malignant new growth by means of a cell-free filtrate. J Am Med Assoc 56:198

Thiess AM, Hey W, Zeller H (1973) Zur Toxikologie von Dichlordimethyläther – Verdacht auf kanzerogene Wirkung auch beim Menschen. Zentralbl Arbeitsmed 23:97

Volkmann R (1875) Über Teer-, Paraffin- und Rußkrebs. Beitrag zur Chirurgie. Breitkopf and Hödel, Leipzig

Wagner JC, Sleggs CA, Marchaud P (1960) Diffuse pleural mesothelioma and asbestos exposure in North-Western Cape Province. Br J Industr Med 17:260

Yamagiwa K, Ichikawa K (1915) Über die künstliche Erzeugung von Papillom. Verh Jpn Pathol Ges 5:142

Validity of Short-Term Tests to Detect Carcinogenic Chemicals

H. Greim, U. Andrae, W. Göggelmann, L. Schwarz, and K. H. Summer

Introduction

Recent advances in understanding of genetic and molecular mechanisms of chemical toxicity have made possible short-term in vivo and in vitro tests to help evaluate the effect of the numerous chemicals in the human environment. The use of these tests has been extensively discussed (Hollstein et al. 1979). Discussion has focused on the significance of the biological end-points and the capacity for metabolic activation. Further aspects of in vitro test systems have received less attention, although they might strongly influence the outcome of the test and its interpretation. One is the balance between the metabolic activation and inactivation of the test compounds; another is the presence in the "artificial" growth media of various components which might alter the cellular response to the toxic agents. Furthermore, the specificity of methods for monitoring toxic effects, especially DNA damage, have not been sufficiently examined.

Because of such complications, many investigators caution the relevance of data obtained from in vitro tests, especially when they do not correlate with those obtained from in vivo experiments. Proper evaluation of such discrepancies requires detailed information on metabolism, pharmacokinetics, mechanism of action of the chemical investigated, and a precise knowledge on the biochemistry of the in vitro test systems applied.

This communication will discuss the relevance of metabolizing systems, of the genetic end-point in mutagenicity systems, and the role of the incubation system in the context of bacterial mutagenicity assays and mammalian cell culture systems, including primary hepatocyte cultures. This should illustrate the potentials and drawbacks of in vitro test systems and contribute to a better understanding of their relevance in risk assessment. It will also help to identify trends in the development of in vitro tests and point out needs for future research.

Metabolic Activation and Inactivation of Chemicals in In Vitro Test Systems

Most of the systems for testing mutagenicity or carcinogenicity using bacteria or mammalian cells have neither sufficient metabolic activation nor inactivation capacities. Since the majority of chemicals causing toxic effects in mammals require metabolic activation, a metabolically active system has to be added. Mostly, a liver microsomal preparation, such as the S9 fraction (postmitochondrial supernatant;

Ames et al. 1975; McCann and Ames 1976; McCann et al. 1975) or the microsomal fraction is used (Malling 1971; Popper et al. 1973; Czygan et al. 1973). In some cases, feeder cells (irradiated cells with inactive genetic systems with high metabolic activities) have been added (Marquardt and Heidelberger 1972). In the most advanced systems, metabolically active cells with intact genetic systems are used. These include either cell lines or primary hepatocytes in which the metabolically activating and inactivating enzymes closely resemble those of the intact liver.

The following discusses advantages and disadvantages in the metabolic capacities of the different test systems:

1. Primary hepatocyte cultures
2. Bacteria
3. Continuous cell lines

Primary Hepatocyte Cultures

The interest in freshly isolated cells as test systems for genotoxicity has largely been focused on hepatocytes since liver is the most active tissue in the metabolism of xenobiotics. The activities of the relevant enzymes in freshly isolated hepatocytes are qualitatively and quantitatively similar to those of the intact liver. However, several activities decrease within a few hours (Schwarz et al. 1979); moreover, it is a major drawback that different activities decrease at different rates. For example, aldrin epoxidase activity representing cytochrome P450-dependent monooxygenases, which occur mainly in liver, decreased to 55% within 12 h and to 8% within 5 days of cultivation (Forster et al. 1986). Similarly, the "hepatic" glucuronosyltransferase (GT) form (GT_2) decreased to 45% at day 5, whereas the GT form which in vivo is present in most tissues (GT_1) remained stable and even increased slightly. Similarly to the GT_1, ethoxyresorufin-O-deethylase (ERDE) activity which represents ubiquitous cytochrome "P448" forms did not decrease over a culture period of 5 days (Forster et al. 1986). In view of the differential decrease of drug metabolizing enzymes in hepatocyte cultures, the results obtained may not only differ quantitatively but also qualitatively with longer incubation times, depending on the enzymes involved in the biotransformation of the chemical under investigation.

So far, attempts to prevent the decrease in the activity of xenobiotic-metabolizing enzymes, specifically of the "hepatic" cytochromes P450, by addition of hormones and certain nutrients to the medium remained unsuccessful. We originally suspected that reactive oxygen species might be involved in the loss of enzyme activity, but addition of antioxidants such as tocopherol or oxygen-metabolizing enzymes remained without effect (Forster et al., unpublished observation).

However, the activity of xenobiotic-metabolizing enzymes in primary hepatocyte cultures may be modulated by other means, i.e., exposure to chemicals which are known to induce these enzymes in vivo. We recently observed (Forster et al. 1986) that benz[a]anthracene (BA) induces the cytochrome P448-dependent deethylation of ethoxyresorufin 12-fold at day 5 of incubation (Fig. 1). Also, exposure to phenobarbital (PB) or pregnenolone-16-α-carbonitrile (PCN) increased this activity 8-fold and 4-fold, respectively. The effects appear to be partially dependent on the presence of dexamethasone, since the degree of induction was lower in the absence of the cor-

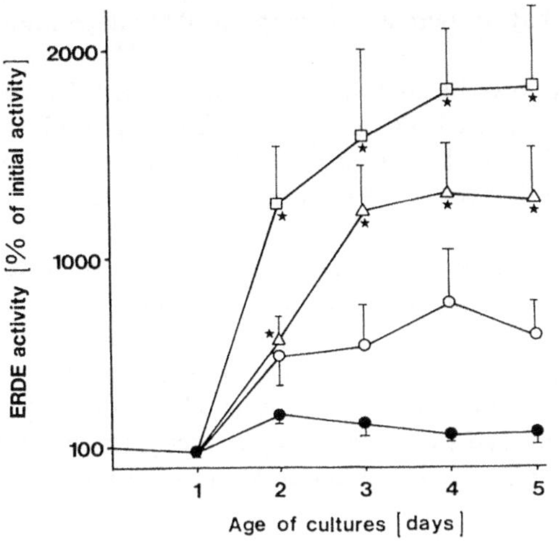

Fig. 1. Induction of ERDE by PCN, PB, and BA in cultured hepatocytes. The initial activity of ERDE was 236 ± 20 fmol/μg of DNA/min. ●, without addition; ○, with 10 μM PCN; △, with 2 mM PB; and □, 15 μM BA. Values represent means (± SE) of 3–5 independent experiments, each performed on duplicate cultures. *, significant differences from control (paired Student's *t* test; $P < 0.05$). For details see Forster et al. 1986

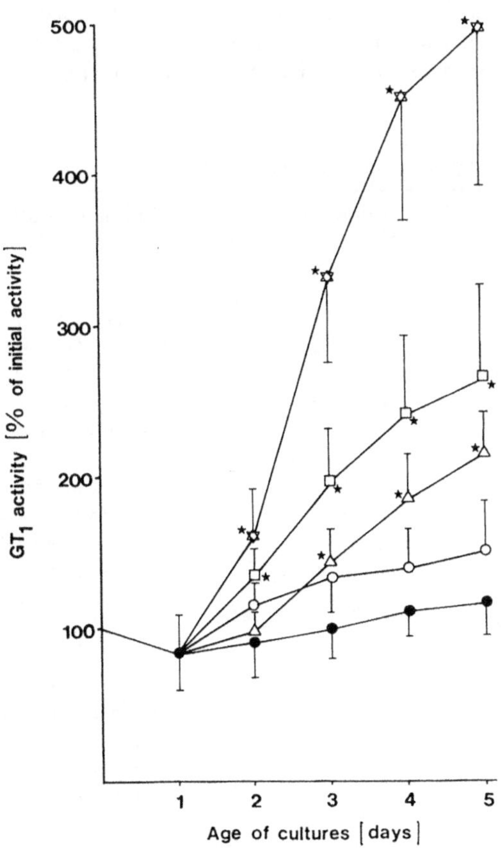

Fig. 2. Induction of 3-hydroxybenzo(a)-pyrene glucuronidation (GT_1) in cultured hepatocytes. The initial enzyme activity amounted to 69 ± 8 pmol/μg of DNA/min. ●, without addition; ○, with 10 μM PCN; △, with 2 mM PB; □, 15 μM BA and ☆, with 15 μM BA and 2 mM PB. Values represent means (± SE) of 3–5 independet experiments, each performed on duplicate cultures. ★, significant differences from control (paired Student's *t* test; $P = 0.05$). For experimental details see Forster et al. 1986

ticosteroid. The inducers, however, failed to increase cytochrome P450-dependent aldrin-epoxidase activity.

The induction of the GT_1 activity followed a pattern similar to that of the cytochrome P448 (Fig. 2). The activity was increased by benz[a]anthracene 2.7-fold, by phenobarbital 2.2-fold, and by PCN 1.5-fold. In contrast to the cytochrome P450-dependent aldrin epoxidase, GT_2 was induced by phenobarbital and to a lesser extent by PCN.

These data demonstrate that certain xenobiotic-metabolizing enzyme activities can be induced in hepatocyte cultures although to very different degrees. All attempts, however, to restore or induce specifically the activity of the "hepatic" cytochrome P450 forms which are particularly prone to decrease with longer incubation times in conventional culture systems have been futile up to now. However, Begue et al. (1984) have reported that rat hepatocytes which are cocultivated with another rat liver epithelial cell type maintain high levels of inducible cytochrome P450 (Begue et al. 1984).

Bacterial Mutagenicity Test Systems

In the Ames test (plate incorporation assay or Salmonella microsomes plate assay) the postmitochondrial supernatant of a liver homogenate (S9 fraction) is used for metabolic activation (Ames et al. 1975; McCann and Ames 1976; McCann et al. 1975; Mattern and Greim 1978). This system, supplied with cofactors of the micro-

Table 1. Drug-metabolizing enzymes mainly involved in inactivation

Enzyme	Location	Cofactor	Typical substrates
Epoxide hydrolases	ER, cytoplasm, nuclear membrane	H_2O	Epoxides
GSH-S transferases	Cytoplasm, ER	GSH	Epoxides, halides, nitrocompounds
Glucuronosyl transferases	ER, nuclear membrane, mitochondria	UDP-glucuronic acid	Phenols, alcohols, carboxylic acids, aromatic amines, amides
Sulfo-transferases	Cytoplasm	PAPS	Phenols, alcohols, aromatic amines
Trans-methylase	Cytoplasm, ER	S-adenosyl-methionine	Catechols, phenols, amines, histamine
Acyl-CoA, glycine transferase	Mitochondria, cytoplasm	Glycine	CoA derivatives of carboxylic acids
N-Acetyl transferases	Cytoplasm	Acetyl-CoA	Aromatic amines, sulfonamides
Esterases	Cytoplasm, ER, mitochondria	H_2O	Aromatic and aliphatic esters, organophosphates, carbamates

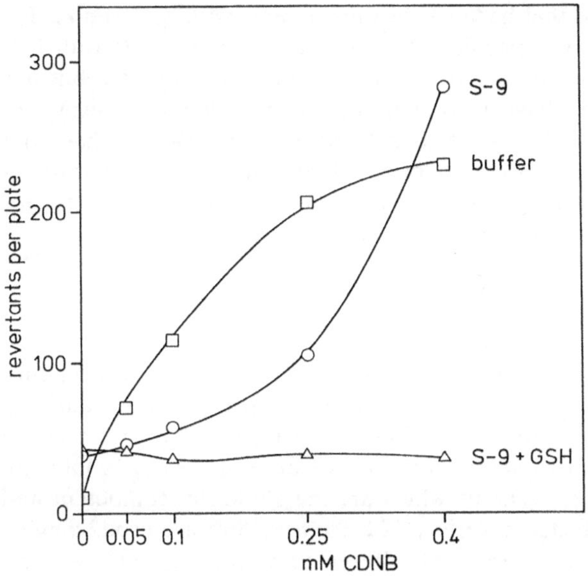

Fig. 3. Modification of chlorodinitrobenzene (CDNB) mutagenicity in the plate incorporation assay by glutathione conjugation. *S. typhimurium* were incubated with CDNB either in the presence of buffer or with post-mitochondrial supernatant (S9) or S9 and 2.5 m*M* glutathione. For details see Summer et al. 1980

somal cytochrome P450-dependent monooxygenase, has a broad capability to metabolically activate most of the chemicals so far tested. In addition, the S9 fraction also contains different inactivating enzymes of microsomal or cytoplasmatic origin (Table 1). Except for the hydrolase, which requires water as cofactor (Ota and Hammock 1980; Guenthner et al. 1981), most of the inactivating enzyme activities are low because of insufficient cofactor supply. However, pretreatment of rats, e.g., with polychlorinated biphenyls, induced cytochrome P450-dependent enzyme activities more than the hydrolase activity. Thus, the metabolic activating enzymes are more active in such test systems than the hydrolase-dependent inactivation processes. The other metabolic inactivation systems, such as sulfotransferases, glucuronosyl transferases, and glutathione-S transferases, are almost inactive. They require cofactors such as sulfate to form 3′-phosphoadenosine-5-phosphosulfate (PAPS; Mulder et al. 1977), uridine-diphosphoglucuronic acid (UDPG; Bock et al. 1981) or glutathione (GSH; Summer et al. 1980), which are not sufficiently present in the S9 fraction.

A consequence of insufficient cofactor availability in the S9 fraction is illustrated in Fig. 3. Chlorodinitrobenzene (CDNB) is a direct mutagen not requiring metabolic activation. It is metabolically inactivated by glutathione conjugation. This enzyme reaction is catalyzed by glutathione-S transferases present in the S9 fraction and the cofactor glutathione. When CDNB is incubated with *Salmonella typhimurium* strains to detect its mutagenicity without S9, a sharp increase in the mutation rate is observed. With S9, the slower increase at low CDNB concentrations is due to the inactivation by glutathione conjugation, provided sufficient amounts of glutathione are present. When high CDNB amounts exhaust glutathione present in the S9, a steep increase in mutagenicity is observed. In the presence of sufficient amounts of glutathione in the S9 fraction, CDNB is inactivated and the chemical is not mutagenic.

Therefore, one can conclude that bacterial test procedures with S9 fractions for metabolic activation are generally specific metabolic activation systems with low metabolic inactivation activities. These systems detect mutagenic potential but not mutagenic potency because they have to be considered to be low or deficient in metabolic inactivation processes. It must be considered, however, that the bacterial strains used in the Ames test possess glutathione and glutathione S-transferase activities (Summer et al. 1980). Although these are low, they may contribute to the inactivation of the chemical, especially when tested at low concentrations.

Continuous Cell Lines

In the search for alternatives to the bacterial test systems, mammalian cells in culture have been examined to see how well they metabolize chemicals. Mammalian cells are either added as "activation systems" to other organisms suitable to detect the genotoxic effect (Marquardt and Heidelberger 1972; Glatt et al. 1981), or they are used as "complete" systems, i.e., systems which are metabolically competent and allow the detection of toxic effects. A variety of cells in culture are used, ranging from freshly isolated cells, through short-lived cultures, to continuous cell lines. Previous observations on metabolic capacity of cells in culture suggested that only freshly isolated cells contain drug-metabolizing enzyme activities closely resembling those found in vivo (Schwarz and Greim 1981; Moldeus et al. 1978; Billings et al. 1977; Decad et al. 1977; Dybing et al. 1979; Vadi et al. 1975; Bates et al. 1981). However, recent results on continuous cell lines indicate otherwise.

The advantage of using continuous cell lines in genotoxicity testing is that they possess a high potential for proliferation and allow the detection of permanent damage, such as mutation or cellular transformation. They are also more suitable for monitoring the appearance of chromosomal damage than are the nonproliferating primary hepatocyte cultures. However, cells in continuous culture have been found to be deficient in the capability to activate premutagens and precarcinogens. This has

Table 2. Expression of xenobiotic metabolizing enzymes in continuous cell lines (Wiebel et al. 1980a, b, 1984a–c)

Enzyme	Substrates	H4IIE	2sFou	C2Rev7	V79	BHK	CHO
Cytochrome P448	a	+	+	–	–	+	–
Cytochrome P450	b	–	+	+	–	–	–
Glucuronosyl transferase 1	c	+	+	+	–	+	+
Glucuronosyl transferase 2	d	(+)	+	+	–	–	–
Phenolsulfotransferase	c	+	+	+	–	–	–
GSH-S transferase	e	+	+	+	+	+	+
Cytochrome C reductase	f	+	+	+	+	+	+
Carboxylesterase	g	+	+	+	+	+	+

Substrates: (a), benzo[a]pyrene; (b), aldrin; (c), 3-hydroxybenzo[a]pyrene; (d), 4-hydroxybiphenyl; (e), 1,2-dichloro-p-nitrobenzene; (f), cytochrome C; (g), α-naphthylacetate prevented their application as self-sufficient systems for genotoxicity testing up to now.

Wiebel and coworkers (1977, 1980a–d, 1984b) have surveyed key enzymes of xenobiotic metabolism in a large variety of cell lines used in toxicological studies. As shown in Table 2 for several representative cell lines, some enzyme activities, e.g., glutathione S-transferase, cytochrome C reductase or carboxylesterase, are strongly retained in continuous cell lines, whereas others, e.g., cytochrome "P450" or phenol sulfotransferase, are readily lost. It is apparent that the different expression of activating and inactivating enzymes in the various cell lines will modify the test results compounding the interpretation in respect to risk estimation. For example, cells such as V79 (derived from Chinese hamster lung) express only certain metabolic activating enzymes and will be relatively sensitive targets for reactive chemicals. In contrast, H4IIE/C3 cells (derived from a rat hepatoma) possess most of the inactivating enzymes and are likely to be more resistent to toxic agents. The different expression of the xenobiotic-metabolizing enzymes in continuous cell lines might, however, also be viewed as an advantage: the presence or absence of specific enzymes offers the possibility to analyse their role in the metabolism of xenobiotics and to clarify the mechanisms of activation.

Recently, there have been some new developments which might radically alter the prospects of continuous cells in genotoxicity studies. Cell lines which were established from H4IIE/C3 cells by Weiss and coworkers and shown to retain liver-specific functions such as gluconeogenesis or production of albumin (Deschatrette and Weiss 1984; Bertolotti 1977; Deschatrette et al. 1979) also express the xenobiotic-metabolizing enzymes of the liver (Wiebel et al. 1980a–d; Wiebel et al. 1984a, b, c; Loquet and Wiebel 1982). In particular, these differentiated lines contain the hepatic cytochrome P450 forms. The following is a list of the evidence for the expression of these cytochrome P450 forms:

1. Substrate specificity
   - epoxidation of aldrin
   - hydroxylation of benzo[a]pyrene (AHH), stimulated by 7,8-benzoflavone, inhibited by SKF 525A
2. Activation of diethylnitrosamine, dimethylnitrosamine
3. Strong activation of aflatoxin B_1
4. Inducibility by phenobarbital
5. Inhibition by monoclonal antibodies against phenobarbital-induced cytochrome P450

(Loquet and Wiebel 1982; Wiebel et al. 1980a, 1984a, b)

Differentiated hepatoma lines such as HF1-4 epoxidize the marker substrate aldrin (Wolff et al. 1979) and hydroxylate benzo[a]pyrene (insensitive to 7,8-benzoflavone; Wiebel et al. 1980). They activate the hepatotoxic agents, dimethylnitrosamine, diethylnitrosamine, and aflatoxin B_1 to their DNA-damaging form (Loquet and Wiebel 1982). Aldrin epoxidase activity is inducible by phenobarbital in these cells (Wiebel et al. 1984c). Finally, aldrin epoxidase activity is specifically inhibited by monoclonal antibodies raised against the phenobarbital-induced monooxygenase of rat liver (Wiebel et al. 1984). As indicated in Table 2 for H4IIE/C3,

2SFou, and C2Rev7 cells, hepatoma lines might contain different forms of cytochrome P450. Thus, there are now cell lines available which are fully competent in the activation (and inactivation) of chemicals in addition to those lines which are characterized by the lack of specific enzyme forms.

Specificity of Methods for Detecting DNA Damage

Many groups of investigators use hepatocytes for in vitro testing of chemicals. Sophisticated analytical methods permit study of a wide variety of mechanisms leading to cytotoxic and genotoxic effects. The use of hepatocytes to investigate cytotoxic mechanisms of action has been reviewed by our group (Schwarz and Greim 1981). Effects of chemicals on membranes, on the synthesis of proteins, RNA and DNA, on energy supply and many other parameters have been studied in isolated hepatocytes. Genotoxic effects of chemicals in these cells can be identified by measuring the induction of DNA strand breaks and DNA repair.

Detection of Unscheduled DNA Synthesis by Audioradiography

The most frequently used method to detect the induction of DNA repair is the so-called "unscheduled DNA synthesis" (UDS) technique. Cells are exposed to the test chemical in the presence of ^{3}H-thymidine. If the compound induces DNA damage subject to excision repair, radioactivity will be incorporated into the DNA during repair synthesis. After exposure, the cells are mounted on glass slides and autoradiographs prepared. The incorporation of radioactivity by DNA repair shows up as silver grains over the nuclei of cells not engaged in replicative DNA synthesis. S-phase cells are easily identified by their heavily labelled nuclei (Williams 1976). Unfortunately, sensitivity and accuracy of the test are affected by a high background of silver grains even in untreated controls. These grains are considered to be the result of thymidine incorporation into the DNA of mitochondria overlaying the nucleus (Lonati-Galligani et al. 1983). Especially when chemicals induce only little DNA repair, it may become impossible to unequivocally differentiate between mitochondrial and DNA repair synthesis in the area of the nucleus.

Cesium Chloride Density Centrifugation to Detect DNA Synthesis

To overcome these problems, the so-called bromodeoxyuridine density-shift method (Pettijohn and Hanawalt 1964) was adopted for use in isolated hepatocytes (Andrae and Schwarz 1981; Rossberger and Andrae 1985). In principle, repair is identified by radioactivity in unreplicated DNA of hepatocytes that were incubated with the test chemical, a radioactive DNA label (^{3}H-deoxycytidine) and a density label (bromodeoxyuridine, BrdUrd). Repaired DNA is separated from replicated, heavily BrdUrd-substituted DNA by ultracentrifugation in cesium salt density gradients. Measurement of repair is not affected by DNA synthesis in S-phase cells or by mitochondrial DNA synthesis. As a consequence, even compounds which induce very little DNA repair synthesis can be identified unequivocally.

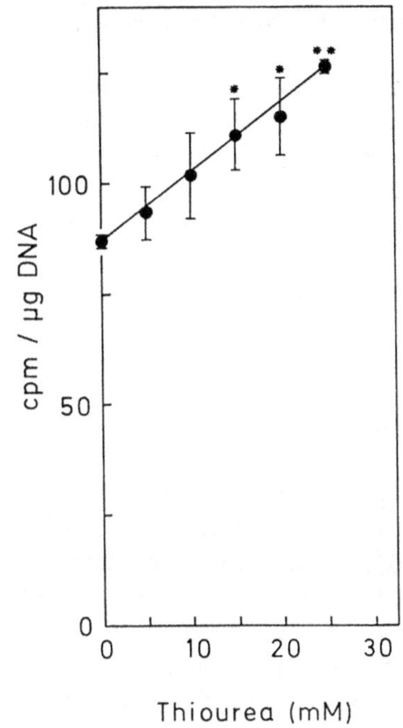

Fig. 4. Repair replication in primary hepatocyte cultures treated with thiourea. Cells were preincubated with FdUrd and BrdUrd, the medium was changed, and the cells were incubated for 18 h with thiourea in the presence of FdUrd, BrdUrd and 10 μCi [^{3}H]dCyd/ml (18 Ci/mmol). Following centrifugation of the isolated DNA in alkaline $CsCl/Cs_2SO_4$ gradients, repair replication was determined as described in Ziegler-Skylakakis et al. 1985. Data represent the means ± SEM from three experiments. *, $P<0.025$; **, $P<0.0005$

An example of the potential of this method, and also of possible pitfalls of repair measurements, is the investigation of whether thiourea which causes tumors in the thyroid and in other organs is genotoxic or not in mammalian cells.

So far, neither thiourea-induced gene mutations nor DNA damage have been observed using bacterial test systems in vitro (McCann et al. 1975; Rosenkranz and Poirier 1979; Simmon 1979). In contrast, thiourea was weakly mutagenic in the intraperitoneal host-mediated assay (Simmon et al. 1979). More recently, Lonati-Galligani et al. (1983), using the autoradiographic method of Williams (1976), detected increased ^{3}H-thymidine labelling of rat hepatocyte nuclei following exposure of the cells to thiourea. They concluded, however, that the increased labelling of mitochondrial DNA overlaying the nucleus mimicked a positive effect; they considered thiourea to be non genotoxic. When the genotoxicity of thiourea in primary rat hepatocyte cultures was reinvestigated using the BrdUrd density-shift method, a linear increase in DNA repair replication at concentrations between 5 and 25 m*M* thiourea was observed (Fig. 4; Ziegler-Skylakakis et al. 1985). Moreover, thiourea was found to be mutagenic in V79 cells (Ziegler-Skylakakis et al. 1985). The results show that maximal sensitivity of a test system is only obtained when the biological end-point measured is highly specific. This is most important when detecting weakly genotoxic chemicals which also exert other effects on cellular metabolism. In the case of thiourea, incorporation of radioactive thymidine into mitochondrial DNA of the hepatocytes also is apparently stimulated by the test compound (Lonati-Galligani et al. 1983). As a consequence, induction of DNA repair is camouflaged by increased mitochondrial DNA synthesis. Both kinds of DNA synthesis cannot be differentiated unequivocally by the autoradiographic technique (UDS) for the detection of DNA repair in hepatocytes.

In conclusion, measurement of chemically induced DNA repair in hepatocyte cultures can be readily used to detect even weakly genotoxic agents, provided the method applied allows a clear discrimination between nuclear and mitochondrial semiconservative DNA synthesis, and repair synthesis. Among the currently available in vitro test systems, the hepatocyte/DNA repair test appears to be most suitable for safety assessment, although additional information on the pharmacokinetics of the chemicals has to be considered before drawing any conclusion about potential hazards.

Role of α-Ketoacids in the Incubation Medium

Pyruvate and other naturally occurring α-ketoacids protect mammalian cells in culture against hydrogen peroxide-induced cytotoxicity (Fig. 5; Andrae et al. 1985) and genotoxicity (Andrae et al., unpublished). We discovered the antioxidant activity of this class of compounds when investigating the effects of different incubation media on the toxicity of reactive forms of oxygen on mammalian cells in vitro. When V79 Chinese hamster cells were exposed to 25 μM H_2O_2 in medium lacking sodium pyruvate, 98% of the cells were killed. Toxicity of H_2O_2 was markedly reduced in the presence of pyruvate. At 12.5 μM H_2O_2, 50% of the cells were killed in the absence

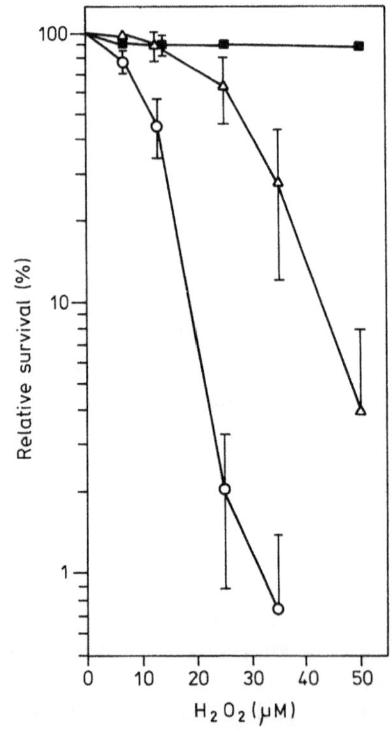

Fig. 5. Effect of pyruvate on the toxicity of H_2O_2 to V79 Chinese hamster cells. 300 cells in BME were exposed to H_2O_2 in the presence or absence of sodium pyruvate for 3 h. The absolute plating efficiency of the control cells not treated with H_2O_2 or pyruvate was 48 ± 16%. Survival of treated cells is normalized to the plating efficiency of the respective control. Each point represents the mean of 4 independent experiments (each on triplicate plates) ± SD. ○, H_2O_2; △, H_2O_2 + 70 μM pyruvate; ●, H_2O_2 + 1 mM pyruvate. For details see Andrae et al. 1985

of pyruvate, but complete survival was observed when 70 μM pyruvate was present during exposure of the cells to H_2O_2. A pyruvate concentration of 1 mM protected completely against even 50 μM H_2O_2, which killed more than 99.9% of the V79 cells in the absence of pyruvate. Other naturally occurring α-ketoacids had similar effects, although to a lesser extent, whereas the corresponding β-ketoacids were ineffective.

The protective action of the α-ketoacids is most likely due to a direct reaction with H_2O_2, resulting in oxidative decarboxylation of the acid, with concomitant decomposition of hydrogen peroxide (Bunton 1949).

The consequences of the presence of pyruvate in cell culture media during experiments on the effects of reactive forms of oxygen in vitro previously have not been recognized. Reactive reduced oxygen species are permanently formed in mammalian cells in vivo and in vitro and have been implicated in the toxicity of numerous xenobiotics (Kappus and Sies 1981). They have been shown to be cytotoxic (Halliwell and Gutteridge 1984), mutagenic (Moody and Hassan 1982; Cunningham and Lokesh 1983), and potentially carcinogenic (Ito et al. 1981). The recognition of the antioxidant activity of pyruvate may help to explain the reasons for the great number of conflicting reports on the effects of H_2O_2 and other reactive forms of oxygen observed in vitro. Moreover, our observations on the effects of pyruvate point out the great importance of careful controls of even minor details in the design of experiments into the toxicity of chemicals in vitro.

Conclusion

At present the applicability and relevance of the various in vitro test systems remain limited due to the fact that biochemistry of the in vitro test systems is little defined and parameters which seem to be negligible to the investigator may greatly influence the outcome of a testing program. For example:

1. Primary hepatocyte cultures rapidly lose metabolizing enzyme activities. They degrade at different rates, the activating enzymes more rapidly than the inactivating ones.
2. False negatives may be created in the standard DNA-repair test in hepatocytes using radioactive precursors to label the newly synthesized DNA. We recently obtained evidence that the collagenase used for isolation of the hepatocyte and the radioactivity introduced into the systems induce DNA-repair activity (Rossberger and Andrae, unpublished results).
3. Most of the mammalian cell lines in culture only possess a very limited capacity to metabolically activate chemicals. Depending on the cell line and its degree of differentiation they express different enzyme activities.
4. The highly standardized *Salmonella typhimurium* strains used in the Ames test contain glutathione and possess glutathione S-transferase activities which may inactivate reactive chemicals leading to false negative results.
5. False positive results may be obtained by the profound differences in the pharmacokinetics between in vitro and in vivo tests. In the intact animal time of exposure of an organ is determined by the half-life of the chemical in the organism, which may be only a few minutes a day when the chemical is given by gavage or injected

once a day. In vitro tests usually involve a constant exposure during the time incubation is maintained.

Due to the many unresolved problems and the various as yet nondefined details which may influence the outcome of the experiments, the application of such cell systems must be considered as a research project rather than a routine experiment. Consequently, defining guidelines especially for the application of mammalian cell systems is premature and would pretend to an as yet nonexisting perfection of the test procedure. In spite of that, in vitro systems have gained and will increasingly gain great importance in studying mechanisms of action and metabolism of chemicals. By this they will provide essential information without using whole-animal studies.

References

Ames BN, McCann J, Yamasaki E (1975) Methods for detecting carcinogens and mutagens with the Salmonella/mammalian microsome mutagenicity test. Mutat Res 31:347–361

Andrae U, Schwarz LR (1981) Induction of DNA repair synthesis in isolated rat hepatocytes by 5-diazouracil and other DNA damaging compounds. Cancer Lett 13:187–193

Andrae U, Singh J, Ziegler-Skylakakis K (1985) Pyruvate and related alpha-ketoacids protect mammalian cells in culture against hydrogen peroxide-induced cytotoxicity. Toxicol Lett 28:93–98

Bates DJ, Foster AB, Jarman M (1981) The metabolism of cyclophosphamide by isolated rat hepatocytes. Biochem Pharmacol 30:3055–3063

Begue JM, Guguen-Guillouzo C, Pasdeloup N, Guillouzo A (1984) Prolonged maintenance of active cytochrome P-450 in adult rat hepatocytes co-cultured with another liver cell type. Hepatology 4:839–842

Bertolotti R (1977) A selective system for hepatoma cells producing gluconeogenic enzymes. Somatic Cell Genet 3:365–380

Billings RE, McMahon RE, Ashmore J, Wagle SR (1977) The metabolism of drugs in isolated rat hepatocytes. Drug Metab Dispos 5:518–526

Bock KW, Bock-Henning BS, Lilienblum W, Volp RF (1981) Release of mutagenic metabolites of benzo(a)pyrene from the perfused rat liver after inhibiton of glucuronidation and sulfation by salicylamide. Chem Biol Interact 36:167–177

Bunton CA (1949) Oxidation of α-diketones and α-keto-acids by hydrogen peroxide. Nature 163:444

Cunningham ML, Lokesh BR (1983) Superoxide anion generated by potassium superoxide is cytotoxic and mutagenic to Chinese hamster ovary cells. Mutat Res 121:299–304

Czygan P, Greim H, Garro AJ, Hutterer F, Schaffner F, Popper H, Rosenthal O, Cooper DY (1973) Microsomal metabolism of dimethylnitrosamine and the cytochrome P-450-dependency of its activation to a mutagen. Cancer Res 33:2983–2986

Decad GM, Hsieh DPH, Byard JL (1977) Maintenance of cytochrome P-450 and metabolism of aflatoxin B_1 in primary hepatocyte cultures. Biochem Biophys Res Commun 78:279–287

Deschatrette J, Weiss MC (1974) Characterization of differentiated and dedifferentiated clones of a rat hepatoma. Biochimie 56:1603–1611

Deschatrette J, Moore EE, Dubois M, Cassio D, Weiss MC (1979) Dedifferentiated variants of a rat hepatoma: analysis by cell hybridization. Somatic Cell Genet 5:697–718

Deschatrette J, Moore EE, Dubois M, Weiss MC (1980) Dedifferentiated variants of a rat hepatoma: reversion analysis. Cell 19:1043–1051

Dybing E, Soderlund E, Timm-Haug L, Thorgeirsson SS (1979) Metabolism and activation of 2-acetylaminofluorene in isolated rat hepatocytes. Cancer Res 39:3268–3275

Forster U, Luippold G, Schwarz LR (1986) Induction of monooxygenase and UDP-glucuronosyltransferase activities in primary cultures of rat hepatocytes. Drug Metab Dispos 14:353–360

Glatt HR, Bilting R, Platt KL, Oesch F (1981) Improvement of the correlation of bacterial mutagenicity with carcinogenicity of benzo(a)pyrene and four of its major metabolites by activation with intact liver cells instead of cell homogenates. Cancer Res 41:270–277

Greim H, Andrae U, Göggelmann W, Hesse S, Schwarz LR, Summer KH (1982) Threshold levels in toxicology: significance of inactivation mechanisms. In: Snyder, Parke, Kocsis, Jollow, Gibson, Witmer (eds) Biological reactive intermediates-II, part B. Plenum, New York, pp 1389–1398

Guenthner TM, Hammock BD, Vogel U, Oesch F (1981) Cytosolic and microsomal epoxide hydrolases are immunologically distinguishable from each other in the rat and mouse. J Biol Chem 256:3163–3166

Halliwell B, Gutteridge JMC (1984) Oxygen toxicity, oxygen radicals, transition metals and disease. Biochem J 219:1–14

Hollstein M, McCann J, Angelosanto FA, Nichols WW (1979) Short-term tests for carcinogens and mutagens. Mutat Res 65:133–226

Ito A, Watanabe H, Naito M, Naito Y (1981) Induction of duodenal tumors in mice by oral administration of hydrogen peroxide. Gann 72:174–175

Kappus H, Sies H (1981) Toxic drug effects associated with oxygen metabolism: redox cycling and lipid peroxidation. Experientia 37:1233–1241

Lonati-Galligani M, Lohman PHM, Berends F (1983) The validity of the autoradiographic method for detecting DNA repair synthesis in rat hepatocytes in primary culture. Mutat Res 113:145–160

Loquet C, Wiebel FJ (1982) Geno- and cytotoxicity of nitrosamines, aflatoxin B_1, and benzo[a]-pyrene in continuous cultures of rat hepatoma cells. Carcinogenesis 3:1213–1218

Malling HV (1971) Dimethylnitrosamine: formation of mutagenic compounds by interaction with mouse liver microsomes. Mutat Res 13:425–429

Marquardt H, Heidelberger D (1972) Influence of "feeder cells" and inducers and inhibitors of microsomal mixed-function oxidase on hydrocarbon-induced malignant transformation of cells derived from C3H mouse prostate. Cancer Res 32:721–725

Mattern IH, Greim H (1978) Report of a workshop on bacterial in vitro mutagenicity test systems. Mutat Res 53:369–378

McCann J, Ames BN (1976) Detection of carcinogens as mutagens in the Salmonella/microsome test: assay of 300 chemicals: discussion. Proc Natl Acad Sci USA 73:950–954

McCann J, Choi E, Yamasaki E, Ames BN (1975) Detection of carcinogens as mutagens in the Salmonella/microsome test: assay of 300 chemicals. Proc Natl Acad Sci USA 72:5135–5139

McQueen CA, Williams GM (1983) The use of cells from rat, mouse, hamster, and rabbit in the hepatocyte primary culture/DNA-repair test. Ann NY Acad Sci 407:119–130

Moldeus P, Högberg J, Orrenius S (1978) Isolation and use of liver cells. Methods Enzymol 52:60–71

Moody CS, Hassan HM (1982) Mutagenicity of oxygen free radicals. Proc Natl Acad Sci USA 79: 2855–2859

Mulder GJ, Henson JA, Nelson WL, Thorgeirsson SS (1977) Role of sulfotransferase from rat liver in the mutagenicity of N-hydroxy-2-acetylamino fluorene in *Salmonella typhimurium.* Biochem Pharmacol 26:1356–1358

Ota K, Hammock BD (1980) Cytosolic and microsomal epoxide hydrolases: differential properties in mammalian liver. Science 207:1479–1481

Pettijohn DE, Hanawalt PC (1964) Evidence for repair replication of ultraviolet damaged DNA in bacteria. J Mol Biol 9:395–410

Popper H, Czygan P, Greim H, Schaffner F, Garro AJ (1973) Mutagenicity of primary and secondary carcinogens altered by normal and induced hepatic microsomes. Proc Soc Exp Biol Med 142:727–729

Rosenkranz HS, Poirier LA (1979) Evaluation of the mutagenicity and DNA modifying activity of carcinogens and non-carcinogens in microbial systems. JNCI 62:873–892

Rossberger S, Andrae U (1985) DNA repair synthesis induced by N-hydroxyurea, acetohydroxamic acid, and N-hydroxyurethane in primary rat hepatocyte cultures: comparative evaluation using the autoradiographic and the bromodeoxyuridine density-shift method. Mutat Res 145:201–207

Schwarz LR, Greim H (1981) Isolated hepatocytes: An analytical tool in hepatotoxicology. In: Berk PD, Chalmers TC (eds) Frontiers in liver disease. Thieme-Stratton, Stuttgart

Schwarz LR, Götz R, Wolff T, Wiebel FJ (1979) Monooxygenase and glucuronosyltransferase activities in short term cultures of isolated rat hepatocytes. FEBS Lett 98:203–206
Simmon VF (1979) In vitro mutagenicity assays of chemical carcinogens and related compounds with *Salmonella typhimurium*. JNCI 62:893–899
Simmon VF, Rosenkranz HS, Zeiger E, Poirier LA (1979) Mutagenic activity of chemical carcinogens and related compounds in the intraperitoneal host-mediated assay. JNCI 62:911–918
Sina JF, Bean CL, Dysart GR, Taylor VI, Bradley MO (1983) Evaluation of the alkaline elution/rat hepatocyte assay as a predictor of carcinogenic/mutagenic potential. Mutat Res 113:357–391
Summer K-H, Wiebel FJ (1981) Glutathione and glutathione S-transferase activities of mammalian cells in culture. Toxicol Lett 9:409–413
Summer K-H, Göggelmann W, Greim H (1980) Glutathione and glutathione S-transferase in the Salmonella mammalian-microsome mutagenicity test. Mutat Res 70:269–278
Vadi H, Moldeus P, Capdevila J, Orrenius S (1975) The metabolism of benzo[a]pyrene in isolated rat cells. Cancer Res 35:2083–2091
Wiebel FJ, Singh J (1980) Monooxygenase and UDP-glucuronyltransferase activities in established cell cultures. Arch Toxicol 44:85–97
Wiebel FJ, Brown S, Waters HL, Selkirk JK (1977) Activation of xenobiotics by monooxygenases: cultures of mammalian cells as analytical tool. Arch Toxicol 39:133–148
Wiebel FJ, Lambiotte M, Summer KH, Wolff T (1980a) Established cell cultures as model systems for carcinogen metabolism. In: Pullman B, Ts'o POP, Gelboin H (eds) Carcinogenesis: fundamental mechanisms of environmental effects. Reidel, Dordrecht, pp 347–361
Wiebel FJ, Schwarz LR, Goto T (1980b) Mutagen-metabolizing enzymes in mammalian cell cultures: possibilities and limitations for mutagenicity screening. In: Norpoth K, Garner RC (eds) Short-term mutagenicity test systems in detecting carcinogens. Springer, Berlin Heidelberg New York, pp 209–225
Wiebel FJ, Singh J, Schindler E, Summer KH (1980c) UDP-Glucuronosylphenol-, sulfo-, and glutathione S-transferase activities of mammalian cells in permanent culture. Toxicology 17:123–126
Wiebel FJ, Wolff T, Lambiotte M (1980d) Presence of cytochrome P-450- and cytochrome P-448-dependent monooxygenase functions in hepatoma cell lines. Biochem Biophys Res Commun 94:466–472
Wiebel FJ, Kiefer F, Park SS, Gelboin HV (1983) Expression of polycyclic aromatic hydrocarbon-inducible and phenobarbital-inducible monooxygenases in continuous hepatoma cell cultures. Naunyn-Schmiedebergs Arch Pharmacol [Suppl] 322:R110
Wiebel FJ, Kiefer F, Murdia US (1984a) Phenobarbital induces cytochrome P-450- and cytochrome P-448-dependent monooxygenases in rat hepatoma cells. Chem Biol Interact 52:151–162
Wiebel FJ, Park SS, Kiefer F, Gelboin HV (1984b) Expression of cytochromes P-450 in rat hepatoma cells. Analysis by monoclonal antibodies specific for cytochromes P-450 from rat liver induced by 3-methylcholanthrene or phenobarbital. Eur J Biochem 145:455–462
Wiebel F, Lambiotte M, Singh J, Summer KH, Wolff T (1984c) Expression of carcinogen-metabolizing enzymes in continuous cultures of mammalian cells. In: Greim H, Jung R, Kramer M, Marquardt H, Oesch F (eds) Biochemical basis of chemical carcinogenesis. Raven, New York, pp 77–88
Williams GM (1976) Carcinogen-induced DNA repair in primary rat liver cell cultures: a possible screen for chemical carcinogens. Cancer Lett 1:231–236
Williams GM (1977) The detection of chemical carcinogenesis by unscheduled DNA synthesis in rat liver primary cell cultures. Cancer Res 37:1845–1851
Wishart GJ (1978) Functional heterogenicity of UDP-Glucuronosyl-transferase as indicated by its differential development and inducibility by glucocorticoids. Demonstration of two groups within the enzyme's activity towards twelve substrates. Biochem J 174:485–489
Wolff T, Deml W, Wanders H (1979) Aldrin epoxidation, a highly sensitive indicator specific for cytochrome P-450-dependent mono-oxygenase activities. Drug Metab Dispos 7:301–305
Wolff T, Greim H, Huang MT, Miwa GT, Lu AYH (1980) Aldrin epoxidation catalyzed by purified rat-liver cytochromes P-450 and P-448. Eur J Biochem 111:545–551
Ziegler-Skylakakis K, Rossberger S, Andrae U (1985) Thiourea induces DNA repair synthesis in primary rat hepatocyte cultures and gene mutations in V79 Chinese hamster cells. Arch Toxicol 58:5–9

Preneoplastic Lesions as Indicators of the Carcinogenic Risk Caused by Chemicals

P. BANNASCH, H. ENZMANN, and H. ZERBAN

Introduction

The evaluation of the carcinogenic potential of chemical compounds depends mainly on the histological demonstration of manifest malignant neoplasia induced in whole animals up to the present. A great disadvantage of this approach is the long lag period in the development of neoplasms produced with chemicals. In order to overcome this drawback, many efforts have been made to detect early biochemical or morphological lesions which might be specific for carcinogens. A vast variety of short-term tests have been carried out in vitro using bacteria, mammalian cell cultures, or isolated hepatocytes (see Greim et al., this volume). These tests provided valuable information about the interactions of many chemicals with various cellular constituents, including macromolecules such as DNA or proteins, but they did not allow an unequivocal prediction of the carcinogenic potential of the respective compounds in whole animals. This unfavorable situation is not only due to the fact that many important parameters such as the absorption, distribution throughout the body, and possible excretion of foreign compounds cannot be studied in the in vitro systems; it is also a reflection of our persistent lack of knowledge of the essential primary event in neoplastic cell transformation. Under these conditions, the detection of phenotypically altered preneoplastic cell populations in various tissues has gained much attention during the past two decades (Bannasch 1984; Carter 1984). In a number of laboratories, systematic studies of the preneoplastic lesions in animal models permitted a distinction between different stages of the carcinogenic process, and led to the recommendation of short-term whole-animal bioassays for carcinogens (cf. Goldsworthy and Pitot 1985b; Pereira and Stoner 1985; Bannasch 1986; Moore and Kitagawa 1986).

The preneoplastic lesions show characteristic cellular changes which have been analysed using conventional light and electron microscopy, enzyme cytochemistry, immunohistochemistry, morphometry, and biochemical microanalysis in some tissues, particularly in rodent liver. The altered cell populations usually form well-defined foci (Fig. 1) which may appear weeks and months prior to the development of certain tumor types in the target tissue of the carcinogen.

The definition of preneoplasia has to include prestages of both benign and malignant neoplasms, especially since many observations suggest that benign tumors are often nothing but intermediate stages in the development of malignant neoplasms. Hence, "preneoplasia" is not identical to "precancer." At the histological level, preneoplastic lesions may be defined as phenotypically altered cell populations which have no obvious neoplastic nature, but have a certain probability of progressing to

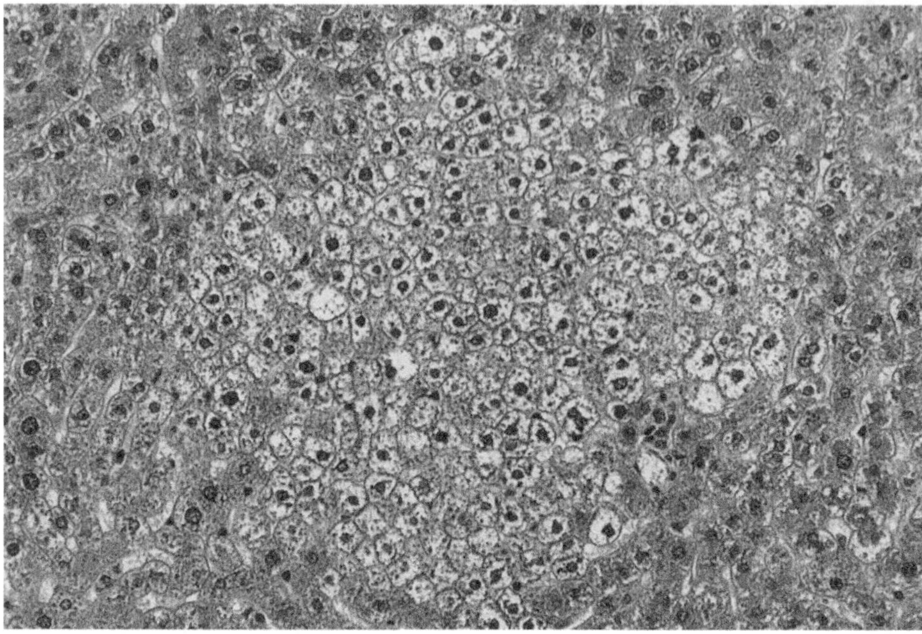

Fig. 1. Preneoplastic clear cell focus induced in rat liver with N-nitrosomorpholine. H&E, × 230

benign or malignant tumors (Bannasch 1986). Theoretically, such a lesion might consist of definitive tumor cells which are only prevented from growing "autonomously" by superordinate mechanisms residing outside the transformed cells, such as the frequently postulated microenvironmental factors or influences of the immune system. On the other hand, preneoplastic lesions might also be composed of cells which are phenotypically altered by the carcinogenic agent, but lack important properties of the final tumor cells. Numerous recent findings suggest that certain types of focal lesions preceding the development of tumors do indeed consist of preneoplastic cells which are only fully transformed after additional intracellular changes (Bannasch 1984). We have to admit, however, that other types of focal lesions may also contain neoplastic cells which might be mixed with preneoplastic cells or even occupy the whole lesion. Thus, the definition of preneoplasia used in this chapter refers to the histological and not necessarily to the cytological level.

Phenotypic Patterns of Preneoplastic Lesions

Hepatic Preneoplasia

Hepatic preneoplasia has been studied most extensively, especially in rats and mice (Bannasch et al. 1984; Farber 1984; Scherer 1984; Ward 1984; Weinbren 1984; Goldsworthy and Pitot 1985b; Pereira and Stoner 1985; Bannasch 1986; Moore and

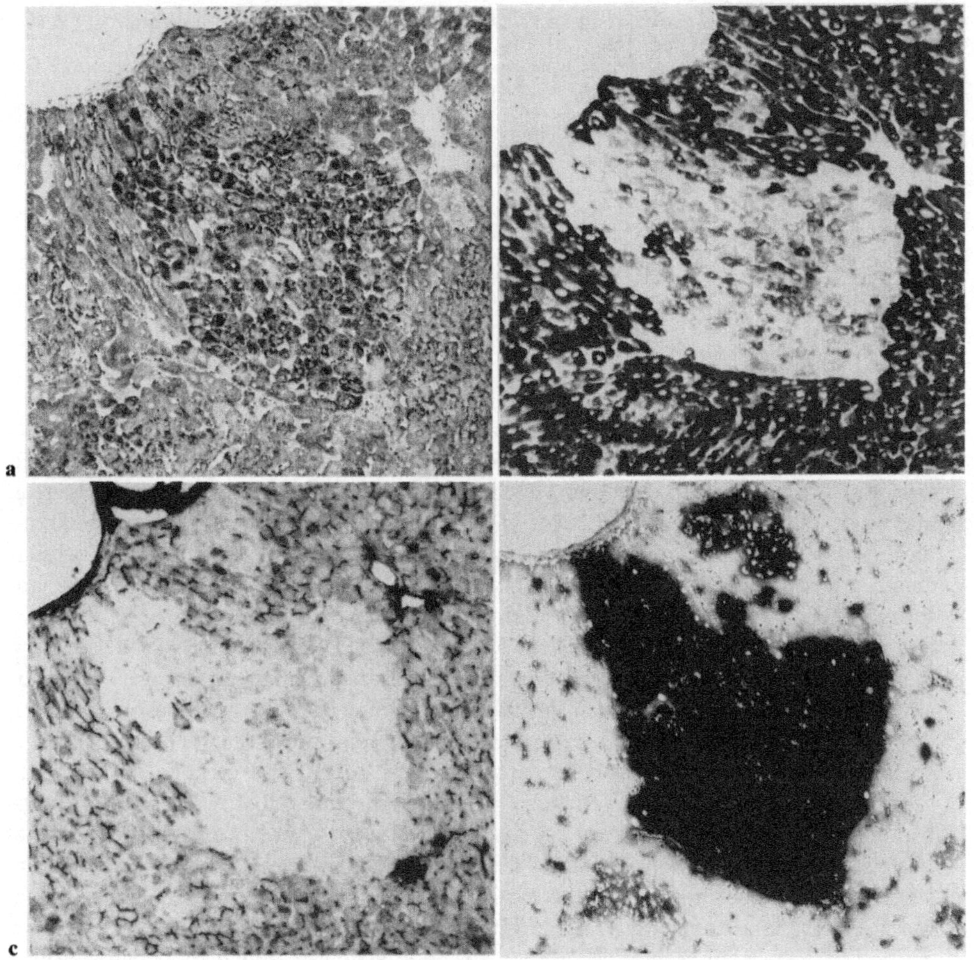

Fig. 2a–d. Serial sections through a preneoplastic glycogen storage focus induced in rat liver with N-nitrosomorpholine. **a** Demonstration of glycogen by the PAS reaction. **b** Decreased activity of glucose-6-phosphatase (lead salt method). **c** Decreased activity of adenosinetriphosphatase (lead salt method). **d** Increased activity of glucose-6-phosphate dehydrogenase (tetrazolium salt method). All parts, × 70

Kitagawa 1986). A turning point for studying early stages of hepatocarcinogenesis was the finding that treatment of rats with nitrosamines produced clear or acidophilic cell foci (Fig. 1) which were characterized by an excessive storage of glycogen (Bannasch and Müller 1964) and often also by a reduction in the activity of the microsomal enzyme glucose-6-phosphatase (Gössner and Friedrich-Freksa 1964), as demonstrated by cytochemical methods (Fig. 2a, b). Similar foci have occasionally been observed in human livers, as a rule in combination with benign or malignant hepatic tumors (for references see Bannasch et al. 1984). Using a laser dissection technique and biochemical micromethods, we were recently able to show that the foci induced

Table 1. Morphological phenotype and classification of foci of altered hepatocytes (from Bannasch 1986)

Type of focus	Glycogen	SER	RER/ ribosomes	Mitosis
Clear cell foci	+ + +	+	+	+
Acidophilic cell foci	+ + +	+ +(+)	+	+
Intermediate cell foci	+ +	+(+)	+ +	+ +
Tigroid cell foci	(+)	+(+)	+ +(+)	+ +(+)
Basophilic cell foci	–	–	+ + +	+ + +
Mixed cell foci	Mixed	Mixed	Mixed	Mixed

in rat liver with N-nitrosomorpholine (NNM) store on average 100% more glycogen than the normal liver parenchyma (Klimek et al. 1984). From light and electron microscopic investigations of a series of experiments in which rats were treated continuously or over short periods (stop experiments) with NNM, a sequence of cellular changes has been inferred which leads from the clear and acidophilic hepatocytes storing glycogen in excess (glycogenosis) to basophilic hepatoma cells poor in glycogen, but rich in ribosomes (Bannasch and Müller 1964; Bannasch 1968). This developmental sequence has also been observed during hepatocarcinogenesis induced in rats by a number of other chemicals, such as diethylnitrosamine, dimethylaminoazobenzene, or thioacetamide (Bannasch et al. 1980), and has been adopted for the classification of specific hepatocellular lesions in rats among which "foci of altered hepatocytes" were separated from expansively growing "neoplastic nodules" by two working groups (Squire and Levitt 1975; Stewart et al. 1980). Recently, we proposed a somewhat more sophisticated nomenclature for the focal lesions (Table 1) which takes into consideration that a certain type of the basophilic focus, called "tigroid cell focus" (Bannasch et al. 1985a) apparently differs in many respects from the basophilic foci described earlier (Bannasch et al. 1985c). Preneoplastic foci which show cytomorphological changes similar to those of the rat have also been detected in other species including primates (Bannasch 1983; Ward 1984; Vesselinovitch and Michailovich 1983).

The obvious cellular heterogeneity of the preneoplastic liver lesions has triggered a controversial debate on the significance of the different cellular phenotypes for the process of carcinogenesis (e.g., Bannasch et al. 1980; Farber 1980; Emmelot and Scherer 1980; Pitot and Sirica 1980; Williams 1980; Kunz et al. 1983; Peraino et al. 1984). For example, Peraino and colleagues felt that each of the diverse phenotypes might represent the result of a specific set of cellular changes, and that the early appearing foci do not evolve through progressively more deviated forms into tumors. However, the concept of a sequential phenotypic conversion of the altered hepatocytes, which we have been pursuing for a number of years, has been further substantiated by studies of the proliferation kinetics (Zerban et al. 1985) and the behavior of the number and size of the different cell populations emerging during hepatocarcinogenesis which was induced by a 7-week treatment with NNM (Enzmann and Bannasch 1986). As demonstrated by the incorporation of ^{3}H-thymidine, the early

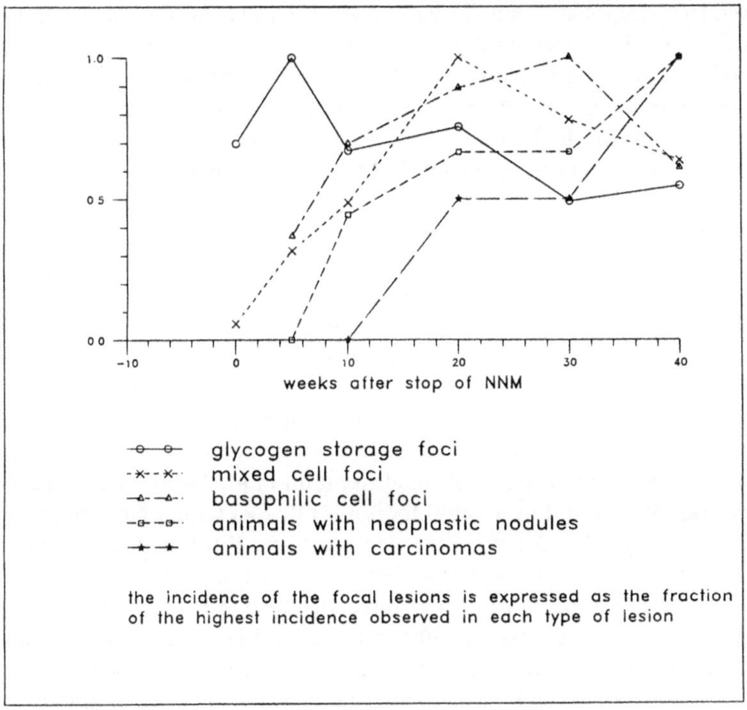

Fig. 3. Sequence of preneoplastic and neoplastic lesions induced in rat liver by a 7-week treatment with N-nitrosomorpholine (120 mg/l drinking water) as studied morphometrically from the end of treatment (0) up to 40 weeks after cessation

appearing clear or acidophilic glycogen storage foci show a slightly increased proliferation, but they do not differ significantly in their growth from the normal liver parenchyma of untreated controls. However, a pronounced and steadily increasing cell proliferation is linked with the appearance of mixed and basophilic cell populations in foci, nodules, and carcinomas. These findings are consistent with the results of morphometric studies of the volume of the different types of foci. Glycogen storage foci were the smallest, basophilic cell foci the largest focal lesions. All foci showed an increase in size with time. This was minimal, however, for the glycogen storage foci and maximal for the basophilic foci. When the number of foci was determined from the end of treatment up to 40 weeks after cessation, predominantly glycogen storage foci and only some mixed cell foci were counted at the beginning (Fig. 3). During the following weeks we observed a temporary increase in the number of mixed cell foci and a progressive decrease in the number of glycogen storage foci. A few basophilic foci appeared for the first time 5 weeks after stop. Later on, there was an increase in the number of basophilic and a decrease in the number of mixed cell foci, the latter starting 20 weeks after stop of treatment. The increase in the number of glycogen storage foci was due to the appearance of small foci of this phenotype. However, the increase in the total number of mixed and basophilic cell foci was not related to an increase of small foci of these phenotypes. On the contrary, the number of small mixed and basophilic cell foci was reduced when the incidence of larger lesions of this phenotype increased. At the same time neoplastic nodules and hepatocellular carcinomas developed. These results suggest that the phenotypic heterogeneity in preneoplastic foci to a large extent reflects different stages in an ordered sequence of cellular changes during hepatocarcinogenesis (Enzmann and Bannasch 1986).

In addition to the alterations discussed so far, a large number of other cellular changes have been described as "negative" or "positive markers," respecticvely, for the carcinogen-induced focal lesions (Peraino et al. 1983; Farber 1984; Scherer 1984; Bannasch 1986; Moore and Kitagawa 1986). Examples of enzymes which frequently show a decreased activity such as glucose-6-phosphatase are the membrane-bound adenosine triphosphatase (Fig. 2c; Schauer and Kunze 1968; Scherer 1984), acid and alkaline nucleases (Taper et al. 1971, 1983), the glycogen phosphorylase (Scherer and Emmelot 1976; Hacker et al. 1982), and the adenylate cyclase which has a central regulatory function in cellular metabolism (Ehemann et al. 1986). An increased activity or content has been found in many (albeit not all) foci with γ-glutamyltranspeptidase (γ-GT; Kalengayi and Desmet 1975; Hanigan and Pitot 1985), DT diaphorase (Schor et al. 1978), glucose-6-phosphate dehydrogenase (Fig. 2d; Hacker et al. 1982; Klimek et al. 1984), a number of other dehydrogenases (Moore et al. 1986a), epoxide hydrolase (Enomoto et al. 1981; Kuhlmann et al. 1981), uridine-diphosphate-glucuronyltransferase (Fischer et al. 1983; Sato et al. 1984), various isoenzymes of cytochrome P450 (Schulte-Hermann et al. 1984; Buchmann et al. 1985), and glutathione transferases (Sato et al. 1984; Buchmann et al. 1985). Moreover, some other functional alterations have been described in preneoplastic hepatic foci of the rat, namely, a resistance to experimental hemosiderosis (Williams et al. 1976; Williams and Watanabe 1978), an enhanced glutathione content (Deml and Oesterle 1980), and a loss of lipid peroxidation (Benedetti et al. 1984). The cytochemical changes appearing in focal liver lesions induced with chemicals in mice in some respects differ from those of the rat, but they also show many similarities (Ward 1984; Vesselinovitch et al. 1985; Numoto et al. 1985).

From the variety of cytochemical changes listed we would like to illustrate in some detail alterations in the alternative pathways of carbohydrate metabolism, in which we were especially interested (Bannasch et al. 1984). Recently we discovered a loss of adenylate cyclase activity in the preneoplastic and neoplastic liver lesions (Ehemann et al. 1986). Adenylate cyclase is the superordinate regulatory enzyme of glycogen degradation, since cAMP, which is the product of the adenylate cyclase reaction, activates a cascade of phosphorylation reactions which finally result in the activation of glycogen phosphorylase. Thus, the decrease in adenylate cyclase activity might explain the reduction in glycogen phosphorylase activity which we have shown earlier in glycogen storage foci (Hacker et al. 1982). The disturbance in phosphorylytic glycogen breakdown is usually accompanied by a reduction of the glucose-6-phosphatase activity, while the activity of glycogen synthetase is not altered. Particularly interesting is the finding that the activity of glucose-6-phosphate dehydrogenase, the key enzyme of the pentose phosphate pathway, is markedly increased in the majority of the glycogen storage foci. More detailed quantitative studies of the glucose-6-phosphate dehydrogenase revealed that there is a gradual increase in enzyme activity from the small glycogenotic foci, which show only a tendency to higher values, over the large glycogenotic to the mixed cell foci (Klimek et al. 1984). These results show that among the many biochemical changes in preneoplastic liver lesions, aberrations in carbohydrate metabolism play an important role. Without going into the details, we would like to mention that these metabolic aberrations might even be causally related to the neoplastic transformation of hepatocytes (Bannasch et al. 1984). This concept is supported by the fact that patients suffering from inborn hepatic glycogenosis have an exceedingly high risk of developing liver tumors in adolescence.

However, some reservations concerning the cytochemical findings are indispensable. Observations in different species indicate that the cytochemical pattern of the preneoplastic foci may even be more heterogeneous than their morphology, and is apparently influenced by many factors, such as the dose and duration of the carcinogenic treatment, the localization of the focal lesions within the liver lobule and the age, sex, and strain of the animals (for references see Bannasch 1986). Of particular interest is that the activity of γ-GT, which has been considered to be a reliable indicator of preneoplastic changes in the liver by a number of laboratories (Hanigan and Pitot 1985), may partly or totally be lacking in certain types of preneoplastic foci in rat liver (Butler et al. 1981; Moore et al. 1983b; Rao et al. 1984; Bannasch et al. 1985a). On the other hand, a periportal focal increase in the activity of this enzyme may also occur in rat liver with age (Kitagawa et al. 1980) or after partial hepatectomy (Bone et al. 1985). Two laboratories (Stäubli et al. 1984; Numoto et al. 1984) reported that the hepatocarcinogenic peroxisome-proliferating hypolipidemic agent nafenopin may "suppress" histochemical γ-GT activity in focal hepatic lesions induced by N-2-fluorenylacetamide.

An especially serious problem for the evaluation of preneoplastic cellular changes in the liver of rodents has become more and more evident during the past few years. In various experimental models it was found that most phenotypic "markers" of hepatocarcinogenesis which have been described so far are not stable and may be mimicked by cellular reactions which are not necessarily related to neoplastic transformation. Thus, under certain experimental conditions, foci (or nodules) have been observed which resemble in their phenotype the persistent lesions appearing during hepatocarcinogenesis, but may disappear to a large extent after cessation of treatment. This reversion-linked phenotypic instability will be discussed in the context of the various models of hepatocarcinogenesis. In addition to this phenomenon, a "progression-linked" phenotypic instability which is related to metabolic and morphologic changes during transformation of preneoplastic into neoplastic cell populations has to be taken into consideration (Bannasch et al. 1985c). Thus, when neoplastic hepatic nodules develop from the preneoplastic foci, the glycogen initially stored in excess is gradually reduced. Whereas the activity of the glucose-6-phosphate dehydrogenase, which is already increased in the preneoplastic foci, remains high, there is usually an additional increase in the activity of the glycolytic enzyme glyceraldehyde-3-phosphate dehydrogenase at this stage of hepatocarcinogenesis (Hacker et al. 1982). Comparable metabolic shifts have been observed by Buchmann and colleagues (1985) for some drug-metabolizing enzymes during progression from foci to nodules.

Preneoplasia in Various Nonhepatic Tissues

Before we look closer into the different animal models of hepatocarcinogenesis, it should be mentioned that preneoplastic lesions have also been described in a number of other tissues (for references see Bannasch 1986). They have not been used systematically in the evaluation of carcinogenesis bioassays, but should be studied in more detail in the future. Some examples of such lesions are the long-known cholangiofibrosis of the rat liver (Bannasch et al. 1985b), nodules of atypical cells in the exocrine pancreas (Longnecker et al. 1984; Scarpelli et al. 1985), so-called goblet cell hyperplasia of the bronchial tree (Gusterson 1984), foci of altered enzyme activity in the urothelium (Hicks and Chowaniec 1978; Kunze 1979), and different tubular lesions in the kidney – each of which is apparently the prestage of a certain, cytologically well-defined tumor type (Bannasch et al. 1986; Bannasch and Zerban 1986). Changes in the activity of various enzymes comparable (but not always identical) to those observed in the liver have recently been described in tubular preneoplastic lesions of the kidney (Ohmori et al. 1982; Tsuda et al. 1985, 1986), the exocrine pancreas (Moore et al. 1983c; Bax et al. 1986), and some other tissues (Moore et al. 1986b).

Models of Hepatocarcinogenesis

A comparison of the results hitherto obtained in a number of experimental models of hepatocarcinogenesis is not only hampered by the frequent lack of a clear separation between (preneoplastic) foci and (neoplastic) nodules, but also by the remarkable variation in the experimental approaches in different laboratories (Fig. 4). Only a few "clean" models for carcinogenesis bioassays using preneoplastic hepatic foci have been proposed. The most convincing models are those in which the test compound is administered for a limited period (Bannasch et al. 1982; Williams 1982) and the animals are investigated up to several weeks or months after withdrawal (stop experiment). In an extreme type of stop experiment a single dose is applied to newborn animals (Vesselinovitch et al. 1979; Vesselinovitch and Mihailovich 1983) or to adult animals after partial hepatectomy (Scherer et al. 1972). Frequently, the additional application of phenobarbital has been used to "promote" the "initiated" cells possibly induced by the test compound, either in young animals (Peraino et al. 1981; Cater et al. 1985) or in adult animals after partial hepatectomy (Pitot et al. 1978; Goldsworthy and Pitot 1985b). This approach has been adopted for the so-called "rat liver foci bioassay" (Pereira 1982; Pereira and Stoner 1985). Although the additional application of phenobarbital renders this system more "sensitive," many problematical interpretations are based on this "two-stage model" since most authors imply that the operational distinction between the "initiator" and the "promotor" allows mechanistic explanations (Goldsworthy and Pitot 1985b). However, a controversial discussion is still going on as to whether phenobarbital merely promotes initiated cells or acts in accord with the "initiator" as a weak carcinogen (Rossi et al. 1977; Feldman et al. 1981; Goldsworthy et al. 1984; Ward and Oshima 1985). There is no doubt that the initiation-promotion protocol may help to detect weak carcinogens. It is difficult to accept, however, when compounds that produce hepatic tumors

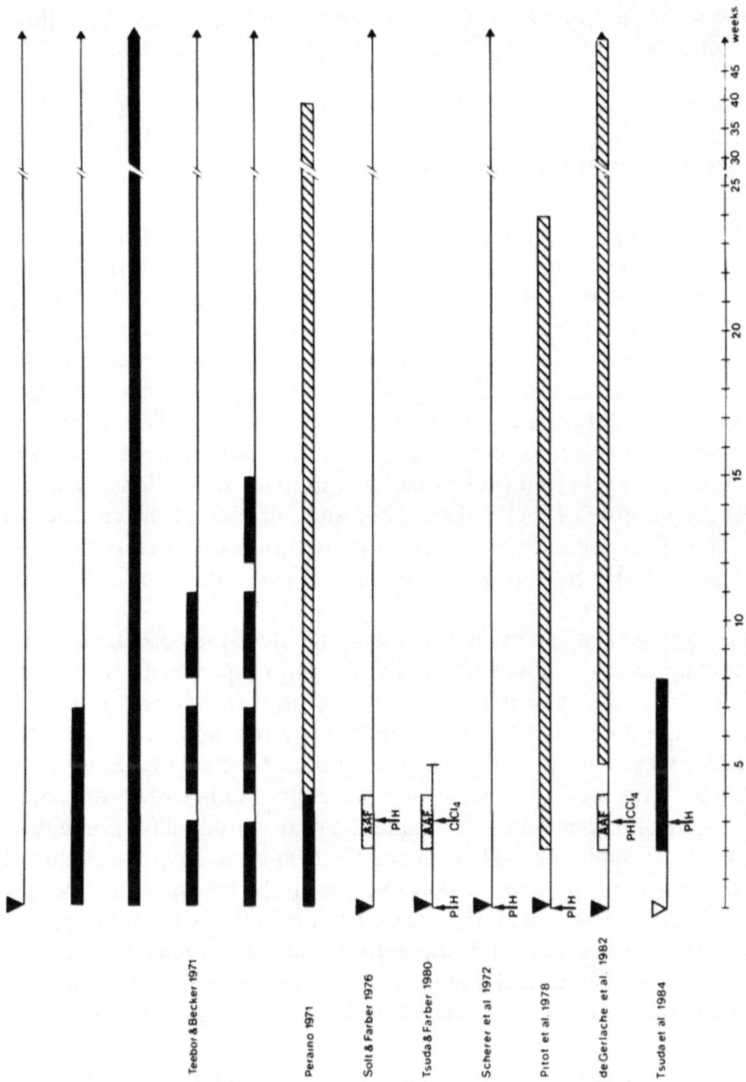

Fig. 4. Schematic presentation of various animal models of hepatocarcinogenesis

without any additional treatment are subsequently grouped with "promotors" if they also enhance the incidence of hepatic tumors initiated by other compounds in the initiation-promotion protocol.

Extremely complex models (Fig. 4) have been developed on the basis of an experiment described by Teebor and Becker (1971) and additional considerations derived from other studies (Solt and Farber 1976; Ito et al. 1980; Tsuda et al. 1980; deGerlache et al. 1982). All of these complex models should be interpreted very cautiously since the additional application of chemicals, some of which are potent carcinogens, hampers the interpretation of the result as long as we know so little about the different effects of the various experimental procedures (Bannasch 1986).

Dose Dependence of Hepatic Preneoplasia

The dose-dependence of hepatic preneoplasia and its relation to the development of hepatocellular carcinomas has been studied by several groups using morphometric methods (Emmelot and Scherer 1980; Pitot and Sirica 1980; Moore et al. 1982; Goldfarb et al. 1983; Kunz et al. 1983; Vesselinovitch and Michailovich 1983; Goldsworthy and Pitot 1985a). The accuracy of measurement of small focal changes in any two-dimensional representation of a three-dimensional process has been considered in great detail by different authors (Fullman 1953; Scherer 1981; Campbell et al. 1982; Pugh et al. 1983; Enzmann et al. 1986). Although the methods used were somewhat varied, all the results indicated that quantitative correlations exist between the size and the number of foci and the dose and duration of the carcinogen treatment. From a statistical point of view there seems to be a good correlation of the dose-time dependence for the early foci and for the later development of liver tumors.

In our own laboratory we studied by morphometric methods the dose-dependence of the sequential cellular changes induced in rat liver by stop experiments with NNM (Moore et al. 1982). The majority of the foci developed after withdrawal of the carcinogen under these experimental conditions (Fig. 5). The first appearance and the frequency of the different lesions investigated proved to depend on the dose of carcinogen administered. With increasing dose of NNM, the number of focal lesions considerably increased, and this was accompanied by an earlier development of mixed and basophilic cell populations. There was no indication of any reversibility of the focal lesions under these experimental conditions. On the contrary, the foci became larger and acquired phenotypic markers closer to neoplasia without further action of the carcinogen. A progressive development has also been revealed by morphometric methods for basophilic foci induced with a single injection of diethylnitrosamine in infant mice (Goldfarb et al. 1983; Vesselinovitch and Mihailovich 1983).

Of particular interest are data concerning the dose-dependence and development of enzyme-altered foci as published by several groups (Emmelot and Scherer 1980; Kunz et al. 1982). Although it has not been taken into consideration so far that a considerable phenotypic instability of enzyme-altered foci and nodules induced by hepatocarcinogens has been observed under certain experimental conditions (Farber 1982, 1984; Moore et al. 1983a; Kitagawa 1971), most of these findings are in accord with the concept of a precursor-product relationship between the foci of altered hepatocytes and hepatic tumors. In this context, it should be mentioned, however, that a direct relationship between focal liver lesions, nodules, and carcinomas has been questioned by some authors (O'Connor and Woodward 1981). Large discrepancies between the number of foci appearing early during hepatocarcinogenesis and final tumor yields are indeed a common finding (Scherer 1984; Emmelot and Scherer 1980; Vesselinovitch and Mihailovich 1983; Kaufmann et al. 1985). This holds espe-

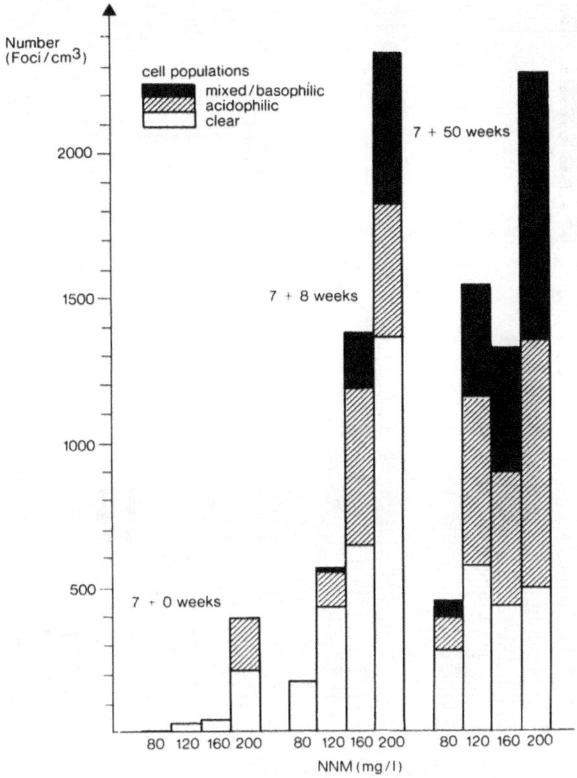

Fig. 5. Dose-dependence of sequential cellular changes in the rat liver as observed in stop experiments with N-nitrosomorpholine in concentrations of 80, 120, 160, and 200 mg/l drinking water for 7 weeks and 8 or 50 weeks after withdrawal of the carcinogen. (After Moore et al. 1982)

cially true for the complex models such as the short-term procedure of Solt and Farber (1976). We used this model giving NNM as "initiator" and analysed the phenotypes of cells from foci and nodules by histochemical methods 1 and 11 weeks after cessation of the AAF treatment (Moore et al. 1983a). Like a number of other authors (for references see Farber 1982; Bannasch 1986), we found that many foci and nodules produced by this regimen regress rapidly (Fig. 6). This has been exemplified morphometrically using the increased activity of glucose-6-phosphate dehydrogenase as a positive marker for foci and nodules. The cause and significance of the regression of foci and nodules varyingly called remodelling (Farber 1978), "reversion" (Williams and Watanabe 1978), "maturation" (Kitagawa 1976), "neodifferentiation" (Farber 1978), or "phenotypic instability" (Moore et al. 1983a) are poorly understood. For an estimation of the extent of phenotypic instability under the experimental conditions of the Solt/Farber system, the recent statement by Farber (1984) is of interest: according to his experience, 95%–98% of the nodular lesions are reversible, while only a few percent persist and may progress to hepatocarcinomas. We, therefore, feel that stop experiments or the continuous application of relatively low doses of the test compound are much more appropriate approaches to study the carcinogenic potential of chemicals using preneoplastic lesions as indicators.

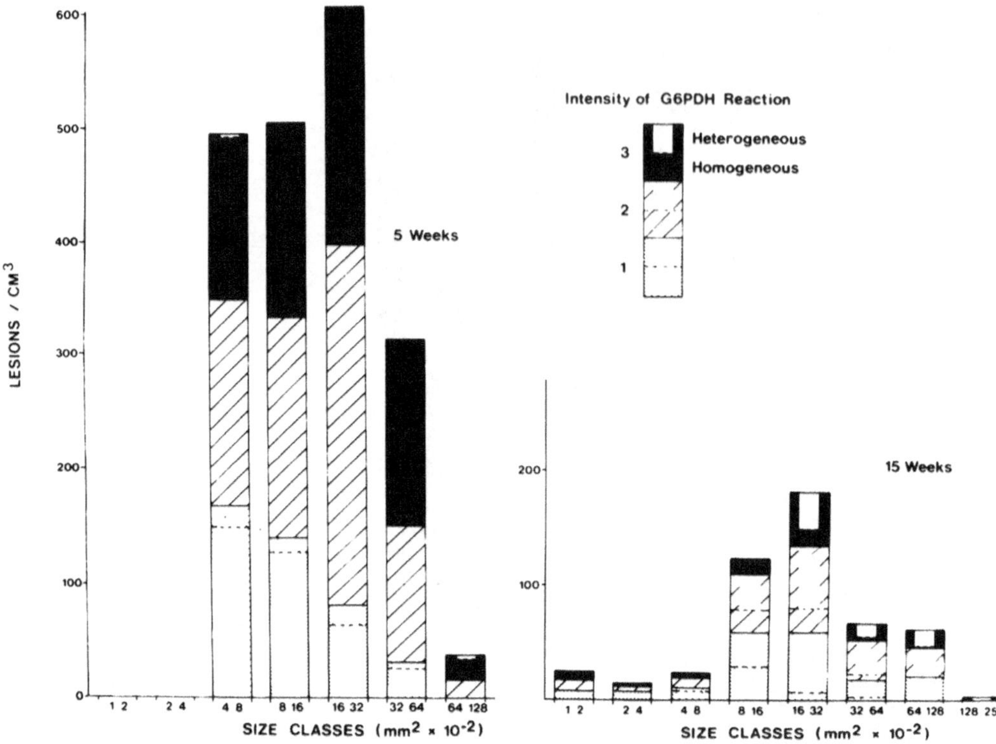

Fig. 6. Number and size distribution of G-6-PDH-positive focal lesions produced in the rat liver according to Solt and Farber, using NNM as an "initiator," 1 and 11 weeks, respectively, after cessation of treatments. (After Moore et al. 1983a)

Usefulness in Bioassays

There appears to be general agreement that the evaluation of bioassays may be improved by consideration of preneoplastic focal liver lesions. If a test compound produces significantly more foci of altered hepatocytes in the treated animals as compared with the concurrent untreated controls, this suggests a carcinogenic potential of the respective chemical. Because of a possible reversion-linked phenotypic instability of the lesions, stop experiments which allow a clear distinction between reversible and persistent, preneoplastic foci should be conducted whenever hepatic foci with a disputed significance appear (Bannasch et al. 1982). Although all hepatocarcinogens investigated so far induced some type of focal hepatic lesion prior to the development of the hepatic tumors, it is not yet clear whether this is always the case. Hence, the absence of hepatic foci after administration of a chemical does not preclude a carcinogenic potential of this compound.

In a recent review, Pereira and Stoner (1985) compared the rat liver foci assay with the strain A mouse lung tumor assay to detect carcinogens. The authors stated that the rat liver foci assay was sensitive to 69% of 54 compounds found to be carcinogenic in long-term bioassays and the strain A lung tumor assay to 54% of 93 carcinogens. None of the 10 compounds found to be noncarcinogenic in long-term bioassays were active in the rat liver foci assay, while seven of 23 noncarcinogens (30%) were active in the lung tumor assay.

The results obtained with the extremely complex models mentioned above have also been reviewed recently. Taking into consideration 80 compounds tested, Parodi et al. (1983) concluded that the "preneoplastic nodules" (foci and nodules were not separated) induced by these complex procedures were more predictive than the Ames test as a statistical trend. However, there was a somewhat better predictability of the "preneoplastic nodules" for liver tumors, as compared with other tumors. It remains to be clarified whether these tests are really acceptable.

Concluding Remarks

The preneoplastic focal lesions identified by cytomorphological and cytochemical methods in a number of tissues, especially in the liver, may well be used as endpoints in carcinogenicity testing. However, many possible pitfalls are evident, and no experimental model is available which might serve as a general test system for the carcinogenic potential of chemicals. Organotropic and cytotropic effects of the chemicals apparently play a crucial role in the production of preneoplastic as well as neoplastic lesions. Thus, preneoplastic lesions in a certain type of tissue do not necessarily predict a similar effect in any other tissue.

Moreover, a certain type of a preneoplastic lesion may not predict all types of tumors potentially developing in this tissue. Nevertheless, the detection of preneoplastic lesions in whole animal studies seems to be more reliable for risk assessment than any known in vitro test. The persistence of specific phenotypic cellular changes induced by a chemical, but independent of its further action after withdrawal, is an important indicator of preneoplastic lesions. Simple experimental systems of the stop type are preferable to complex models, although such simple systems may not fulfill the requirements for a "short-term test." The absence of foci of altered cells after administration of a chemical does not preclude a carcinogenic potential of this compound. However, the detection of persistent foci may considerably improve the evaluation of carcinogenesis bioassays and save both animals and time.

Acknowledgements. We would like to express our appreciation to Dr. Volker Ehemann for the contribution of Fig. 2a–d, and to Kornelia Müller for secretarial help.

References

Bannasch P (1968) The cytoplasm of hepatocytes during carcinogenesis. Light and electron microscopic investigations of the nitrosomorpholine-intoxicated rat liver. Rec Res Cancer Res 19:1–100

Bannasch P (1983) Strain and species differences in the susceptibility to liver tumor induction. IARC Scientific Publications 51:9–38

Bannasch P (1984) Sequential cellular changes during chemical carcinogenesis. J Cancer Res Clin Oncol 108:11–22

Bannasch P (1986) Preneoplastic lesions as end points in carcinogenecity testing. I. Hepatic preneoplasia and II. Preneoplasia in various non-hepatic tissues. Carcinogenesis 7:689–695, 849–852

Bannasch P, Müller HA (1964) Lichtmikroskopische Untersuchungen über die Wirkung von N-Nitrosomorpholin auf die Leber von Ratte und Maus. Arzneimittelforsch 14:805–814
Bannasch P, Zerban H (1986) Renal cell adenoma and carcinoma. In: Jones TC, Mohr U, Hunt RD (eds) Monographs on pathology of laboratory animals, urinary system. Springer, Berlin Heidelberg New York Tokyo, pp 112-139
Bannasch P, Mayer D, Hacker HJ (1980) Hepatocellular glycogenosis and hepatocarcinogenesis. Biochim Biophys Acta 605:217–245
Bannasch P, Moore MA, Klimek F, Zerban H (1982) Biological markers of preneoplastic foci and neoplastic nodules in rodent liver. Toxicol Pathol 10:19–34
Bannasch P, Hacker HJ, Klimek F, Mayer D (1984) Hepatocellular glycogenosis and related pattern of enzymatic changes during hepatocarcinogenesis. Adv Enzyme Regul 22:97–121
Bannasch P, Benner U, Enzmann H, Hacker HJ (1985a) Tigroid cell foci and neoplastic nodules in the liver of rats treated with a single dose of aflatoxin B_1. Carcinogenesis 11:1641–1648
Bannasch P, Benner U, Zerban H (1985b) Cholangiofibroma and cholangiocarcinoma, liver, rat. In: Jones TC, Mohr U, Hunt RD (eds) Monographs on pathology of laboratory animals, digestive system. Springer, Berlin Heidelberg New York Tokyo, pp 52–65
Bannasch P, Zerban H, Hacker HJ (1985c) Foci of altered hepatocytes, rat. In: Jones TC, Mohr U, Hunt RD (eds) Monographs on pathology of laboratory animals, digestive system. Springer, Berlin Heidelberg New York Tokyo, pp 10–30
Bannasch P, Zerban H, Hacker HJ (1986) Oncocytoma, kidney, rat. In: Jones TC, Mohr U, Hunt RD (eds) Monographs on pathology of laboratory animals, urinary system. Springer, Berlin Heidelberg New York Tokyo, pp 49-60
Bax J, Feringa AW, van Garderen-Hoetmer A, Woutersen RA, Scherer E (1986) Adenosine triphosphatase, a new marker for the differentiation of putative precancerous foci induced in rat pancreas by azaserine. Carcinogenesis 7:457–462
Benedetti A, Malvadi G, Fulceri R, Comporti M (1984) Loss of lipid peroxidation as a histochemical marker for preneoplastic hepatocellular foci of rats. Cancer Res 44:5712–5717
Bone III SN, Michalopoulos G, Jirtle RL (1985) Ability of partial hepatectomy to induce γ-glutamyltranspeptidase in regenerated and transplanted hepatocytes of Fischer 344 and Wistar-Furth rats. Cancer Res 45:1222–1228
Buchmann A, Kuhlmann WD, Schwarz M, Kunz HW, Wolf CR, Moll E, Friedberg T, Oesch F (1985) Regulation and expression of four cytochrome P-450 isoenzymes, NADPH-cytochrome P-450 reductase, the glutathione transferase B and C and microsomal epoxide hydrolase in preneoplastic and neoplastic lesions in rat liver. Carcinogenesis 6:513–521
Butler WH, Hempsall V, Stewart MC (1981) Histochemical studies on the early proliferating lesions induced in the rat liver by aflatoxin. J Pathol 133:325–340
Campbell HA, Pitot HC, Potter VR, Laishes BA (1982) Application of quantitative stereology to the evaluation of enzyme-altered foci in rat liver. Cancer Res 42:465–472
Carter RL (ed) (1984) Precancerous States. Oxford University Press, London
Cater KC, Gandolfi AJ, Sipes IG (1985) Characterization of dimethyl-nitrosamine-induced focal and nodular lesions in the livers of newborn mice. Toxicol Pathol 13:3–9
de Gerlache J, Lans M, Taper H, Préat V, Roberfroid M (1982) Promotion of the chemically initiated hepatocarcinogenesis. In: Sorsa M, Vaina H (eds) Mutagens in our environment. Liss, New York, pp 35–46
Deml E, Oesterle D (1980) Histochemical demonstration of enhanced glutatione content in enzyme-altered islands induced by carcinogens in rat liver. Cancer Res 40:490–491
Ehemann V, Mayer D, Hacker HJ, Bannasch P (1986) Loss of adenylate cyclase activity in preneoplastic and neoplastic lesions induced in rat liver by N-nitrosomorpholine. Carcinogenesis 7:567–573
Emmelot P, Scherer E (1980) The first relevant cell stage in rat liver carcinogenesis. A quantitative approach. Biochim Biophys Acta 605:247–304
Enomoto K, Ying TS, Griffin MJ, Farber E (1981) Immunohistochemical study of epoxide hydrolase during experimental liver carcinogenesis. Cancer Res 41:3281–3287
Enzmann H, Bannasch P (1986) Sequential phenotypic conversion of hepatocytes during carcinogenesis. Cancer Lett 30:S67
Enzmann H, Edler L, Bannasch P (1987) Simple elementary method for the quantification of focal liver lesions induced by carcinogens. Carcinogenesis (in press)

Farber E (1978) Experimental liver carcinogenesis: a perspective. In: Remmer H, Bolt HM, Bannasch P, Popper H (eds) Primary liver tumors. MTP Press, Lancaster, England, pp 357–375
Farber E (1980) The sequential analysis of cancer induction. Biochim Biophys Acta 605:149–166
Farber E (1982) The biology of carcinogen-induced hepatocyte nodules and related liver lesions in the rat. Toxicol Pathol 10:197–205
Farber E (1984) Pre-cancerous steps in carcinogenesis. Their physiological adaptive nature. Biochim Biophys Acta 738:171–180
Feldman D, Swarm RL, Becker J (1981) Ultrastructural study of rat liver and liver neoplasms after long-term treatment with phenobarbital. Cancer Res 41:2151–2162
Fischer G, Ullrich D, Katz N, Bock WK, Schauer A (1983) Immunohistochemical and biochemical detection of uridine-diphosphate-glucuronyl-transferase (UDP-GT) activity in putative preneoplastic liver foci. Virchows Arch B [Cell Pathol] 42:193–200
Fullman RL (1953) Measurement of particle sizes in opaque bodies. Trans AIME 197:447–452
Gössner W, Friedrich-Freksa (1964) Histochemische Untersuchungen über die Glucose-6-Phosphatase in der Rattenleber während der Cancerisierung durch Nitrosamine. Z Naturforsch 19b:862–864
Goldfarb S, Pugh TD, Koen H, He YZ (1983) Preneoplastic and neoplastic progression during hepatocarcinogenesis in mice injected with diethylnitrosamine in infancy. Environ Health Perspect 50:149–161
Goldsworthy TL, Pitot HC (1985a) The quantitative analysis and stability of histochemical markers of altered hepatic foci in rat liver following initiation by diethylnitrosamine administration and promotion with phenobarbital. Carcinogenesis 6:1261–1269
Goldsworthy TL, Pitot HC (1985b) An approach to the development of a short-term whole animal bioassay to distinguish initiating agents (incomplete carcinogens), promoting agents, complete carcinogens, and noncarcinogens in rat liver. J Toxicol Environ Health 16:389–402
Goldsworthy T, Campbell HA, Pitot HC (1984) The natural history and dose-response characteristics of enzyme-altered foci in rat liver following phenobarbital and diethylnitrosamine administration. Carcinogenesis 5:67–71
Gusterson BA (1984) Precancerous changes in the lungs and the potential of cells to have modulated phenotypes. In: Carter RL (ed) Precancerous states. Oxford University Press, London, pp 161–184
Hacker HJ, Moore MA, Mayer D, Bannasch P (1982) Correlative histochemistry of some enzymes of carbohydrate metabolism in preneoplastic and neoplastic lesions in the rat liver. Carcinogenesis 3:1265–1272
Hanigan MH, Pitot HC (1985) Gamma-glutamyl transpeptidase – its role in hepatocarcinogenesis. Carcinogenesis 6:165–172
Hicks RM, Chowaniec J (1978) Experimental induction, histology, and ultrastructure of hyperplasia and neoplasia of the urinary bladder epithelium. Int Rev Exp Pathol 18:199–280
Ito N, Tatematsu M, Nakanishi K, Hasegawa R, Takano T, Imaida K, Ogiso T (1980) The effects of various chemicals on the development of hyperplastic liver nodules in hepatectomized rats treated with N-nitrosodiethylamine or N-2-fluorenylacetamide. Gann 71:832–842
Kalengayi MMR, Desmet VJ (1975) Sequential histological and histochemical study of the rat liver during aflatoxin B_1-induced carcinogenesis. Cancer Res 35:2845–2852
Kaufmann WK, Mackenzie SA, Kaufman DG (1985) Quantitative relationship between hepatocytic neoplasms and island of cellular alterations during hepatocarcinogenesis in the male F344 rat. Am J Pathol 119:171–174
Kitagawa T (1971) Histochemical analysis of hyperplastic lesions and hepatomas of the liver of rats fed 2-fluorenylacetamide. Gann 62:207–216
Kitagawa T (1976) Sequential phenotypic changes in hyperplastic areas during hepatocarcinogenesis in the rat. Cancer Res 36:2534–1539
Kitagawa T, Imai F, Sato K (1980) Re-elevation of γ-glutamyl transpeptidase activity in periportal hepatocytes of rats with age. Gann 71:362–366
Klimek F, Mayer D, Bannasch P (1984) Biochemical microanalysis of glycogen content and glucose-6-phosphate dehydrogenase activity in focal lesions of rat liver induced by N-nitrosomorpholine. Carcinogenesis 5:265–268
Kuhlmann WD, Krishan R, Kunz W, Guenthner TM, Oesch F (1981) Focal elevation of liver microsomal epoxide hydrolase in early preneoplastic stages and its behaviour in the further course of hepatocarcinogenesis. Biochem Biophys Res Commun 98:417–423

Kunz HW, Tennekes HA, Port RE, Schwarz M, Lorke D, Schaude G (1983) Quantitative aspects of chemical carcinogenesis and tumor promotion in liver. Environ Health Perspect 50:113–122
Kunz W, Schaude G, Schwarz M, Tennekes H (1982) Quantitative aspects of drug-mediated tumour promotion in liver and its toxicological implications. In: Hecker E, Fusenig N, Marks F, Kunz W (eds) Carcinogenesis – a comprehensive survey. Raven, New York, pp 111–125
Kunze E (1979) Development of urinary bladder cancer in the rat. Curr Top Pathol 67:145–232
Longnecker DS, Wiebkin P, Schaeffer BK, Roebuck BD (1984) Experimental carcinogenesis in the pancreas. Int Rev Exp Pathol 26:177–229
Moore MA, Kitagawa T (1986) Hepatocarcinogenesis in the rat; the effect of the promoters and carcinogens in vivo and in vitro. Int Rev Cytol 101:125–173
Moore MA, Mayer D, Bannasch P (1982) The dose-dependence and sequential appearance of putative preneoplastic populations induced in the rat liver by stop experiments with N-nitrosomorpholine. Carcinogenesis 3:1429–1436
Moore MA, Hacker HJ, Bannasch P (1983a) Phenotypic instability in focal and nodular lesions induced in a short-term system in the rat liver. Carcinogenesis 4:595–603
Moore MA, Hacker HJ, Kunz HW, Bannasch P (1983b) Enhancement of NNM-induced carcinogenesis in the rat liver by phenobarbital: a combined morphological and enzyme histochemical approach. Carcinogenesis 4:473–479
Moore MA, Takahashi M, Ito N, Bannasch P (1983c) Early lesions during pancreatic carcinogenesis induced in Syrian hamster by DHPN or DOPN. I. Histologic, histochemical and radioautographic findings. Carcinogenesis 4:431–437
Moore MA, Tsuda H, Ito N (1986a) Dehydrogenase histochemistry of N-ethyl-N-hydroxyethylnitrosamine-induced focal liver lesions in the rat-increase in NADPH-generating capacity. Carcinogenesis 7:339–342
Moore MA, Nakamura T, Shirai T, Ito N (1986b) Immunohistochemical demonstration of increased glucose-6-phosphate dehydrogenase in preneoplastic and neoplastic lesions induced by propylnitrosamines in F344 rats and Syrian hamsters. Jpn J Cancer Res (Gann) 77:131–138
Numoto S, Furukawa K, Furuya K, Williams GM (1984) Effects of the hepatocarcinogenic peroxisome-proliferating hypolipidemic agents Clofibrate and Nafenopin on the rat liver cell membrane enzymes γ-glutamyltranspeptidase and alkaline phosphatase and on the early stages of liver carcinogenesis. Carcinogenesis 5:1603–1611
Numoto S, Tanaka T, Williams GM (1985) Morphologic and cytochemical properties of mouse liver neoplasms induced by diethylnitrosamine and promoted by 4,4′-dichlorodiphenyltrichloroethane, Chlordane, or heptachlor. Toxicol Pathol 13:325–334
O'Connor CA, Woodward SC (1981) Industry's role in cancer research: anticipating regulatory problems. Regul Toxicol Pharmacol 1:316–334
Ohmori T, Hiasa Y, Murata Y, Williams GM (1982) Gamma glutamyl transpeptidase activity in carcinogen-induced epithelial lesions of rat kidney. Gann 73:543–548
Parodi S, Taningher M, Santi L (1983) Induction of preneoplastic nodules: quantitative predictivity of carcinogenicity. Anticancer Res 3:393–400
Peraino C, Fry R, Staffeldt E (1971) Reduction and enhancement by phenobarbital of hepatocarcinogenesis induced in rat by 2-acetylamino-fluorene. Cancer Res 31:1506–1512
Peraino C, Staffeldt EF, Ludeman VA (1981) Early appearance of histochemically altered hepatocyte foci and liver tumors in female rats treated with carcinogens one day after birth. Carcinogenesis 2:463–465
Peraino C, Richards WL, Stevens FJ (1983) Multistage hepatocarcinogenesis. In: Slaga TJ (ed) Mechanisms of tumor promotion, vol 1. CRC Press, Boca Raton, pp 1–53
Peraino C, Staffeldt EF, Carnes BA, Ludeman VA, Blomquist JA, Vesselinovitch SD (1984) Characterization of histochemically detectable altered hepatocyte foci and their relationship to hepatic tumorigenesis in rats treated once with diethylnitrosamine or benzo(a)pyrene within one day after birth. Cancer Res 44:3340–3347
Pereira MA (1982) Rat liver foci bioassay. J Am Coll Toxicol 1:101–117
Pereira MA, Stoner GD (1985) Comparison of rat liver foci assay and strain mouse lung tumor assay to detect carcinogens: a review. Fund Appl Toxicol 5:688–699
Pitot HC, Sirica AE (1980) The stages of initiation and promotion in hepatocarcinogenesis. Biochim Biophys Acta 605:191–215

Pitot HC, Barsness L, Goldsworthy F, Kitagawa T (1978) Biochemical characterisation of stages of hepatocarcinogenesis after a single dose of diethylnitrosamine. Nature 271:456–458

Pugh TD, King JH, Koen H, Nychka D, Chover J, Wahba G, He YH, Goldfarb S (1983) Reliable stereological method for estimating the number of microscopic hepatocellular foci from their transections. Cancer Res 43:1261–1268

Rao MS, Lalwani ND, Reddy JK (1984) Sequential histologic study of rat liver during peroxisome proliferator [4-chloro-6(2,3-xylidino)-2-pyrimidinylthio]-acetic acid (Wy-14,643)-induced carcinogenesis. JNCI 73:983–990

Rossi L, Ravera M, Repetti G, Santi L (1977) Long-term administration of DDT or phenobarbital-Na in Wistar rats. Int J Cancer 19:179–185

Sato K, Kitahara A, Satoh K, Ishikawa T, Tatematsu M, Ito N (1984) The placental form of glutathione S-transferase as a new marker protein for preneoplasia in rat chemical carcinogenesis. Gann 75:199–202

Scarpelli DG, Rao MS, Reddy JK (1985) Experimental carcinogenesis of exocrine pancreas: animal models, neoplasms, and current understanding of pathogenesis. In: Jones TC, Mohr U, Hunt RD (eds) Monographs on pathology of laboratory animals, digestive system. Springer, Berlin Heidelberg New York Tokyo, pp 224–238

Schauer A, Kunze E (1968) Enzymhistochemische und autoradiographische Untersuchungen während der Kanzerisierung der Rattenleber durch Diäthylnitrosamin. Z Krebsforsch 70:252–266

Scherer E (1981) Use of a programmable pocket calculator for the quantitation of precancerous foci. Carcinogenesis 2:805–807

Scherer E (1984) Neoplastic progression in experimental hepatocarcinogenesis. Biochim Biophys Acta 738:219–236

Scherer E, Emmelot P (1975) Foci of altered liver cells induced by a single dose of diethylnitrosamine and partial hepatectomy: their contribution to hepatocarcinogenesis in rat. Eur J Cancer 11: 145–154

Scherer E, Emmelot P (1976) Kinetics of induction and growth of enzyme-deficient islands involved in hepatocarcinogenesis. Cancer Res 36:2544–2554

Scherer E, Hoffmann M, Emmelot P, Friedrich-Freska H (1972) Quantitative study on foci of altered liver cells induced in the rat by a single dose of diethylnitrosamine and partial hepatectomy. JNCI 49:93–106

Schor NA, Ogawa K, Lee G, Farber E (1978) The use of the D-T diaphorase for the detection of foci of early neoplastic transformation in rat liver. Cancer Lett 5:167–171

Schulte-Hermann R, Roome N, Timmermann-Trosiener I, Schuppler J (1984) Immunocytochemical demonstration of a phenobarbital-inducible cytochrome P-450 in putative preneoplastic foci of rat liver. Carcinogenesis 5:143–153

Solt D, Farber E (1976) New principle for the analysis of chemical carcinogenesis. Nature 263:702–703

Squire RA, Levitt MH (1975) Report of a workshop on classification of specific hepatocellular lesions in rats. Cancer Res 35:3214–3223

Stäubli W, Bently P, Bieri F, Fröhlich E, Waechter F (1984) Inhibitory effect of nafenopin upon the development of diethylnitrosamine-induced enzyme altered foci within the rat liver. Carcinogenesis 5:41–46

Stewart HL, Williams G, Keysser CH, Lombard LS, Montali RJ (1980) Histologic typing of liver tumors of the rat. JNCI 65:179–206

Taper HS, Fort L, Brucher JM (1971) Histochemical activity of alkaline and acid nucleases in the rat liver parenchyma during N-nitrosomorpholine carcinogenesis. Cancer Res 31:913–916

Taper HS, Lans M, deGerlache J, Fort L, Roberfroid M (1983) Morphological alterations and DNase deficiency in phenobarbital promotion of N-nitrosomorpholine initiated rat hepatocarcinogenesis. Carcinogenesis 4:231–234

Teebor GW, Becker FF (1971) Regression and persistence of hyperplastic nodules induced by N-2-fluorenylacetamide and their relationship to hepatocarcinogenesis. Cancer Res 31:1–3

Tsuda H, Farber E (1980) Resistant hepatocytes as early changes in liver induced by polycyclic aromatic hydrocarbons. Int J Cancer 25:137–139

Tsuda H, Lee G, Farber E (1980) Induction of resistant hepatocytes as a new principle for a possible short term in vivo test for carcinogens. Cancer Res 40:1157–1164

Tsuda H, Hasegawa R, Imaida K, Masui T, Moore MA, Ito N (1984) Modifying potential of thirty-one chemicals on the short-term development of γ-glutamyl transpeptidase-positive foci in diethylnitrosamine-initiated rat liver. Gann 74:876–883

Tsuda H, Moore MA, Asamoto M, Satoh K, Tsuchida S, Sato K, Ichihara A, Ito N (1985) Comparison of the various forms of glutathione S-transferase with glucose-6-phosphate dehydrogenase and γ-glutamyl transpeptidase as markers of preneoplastic and neoplastic lesion in rat kidney induced by N-ethyl-N-hydroxyethylnitrosamine. Jpn J Cancer Res (Gann) 76:919–929

Tsuda H, Hacker HJ, Katayama H, Masui T, Ito N, Bannasch P (1986) Correlative histochemical studies on preneoplastic and neoplastic lesions in the kidney of rats treated with nitrosamines. Virchows Arch B [Cell Pathol] 51:385–404

Vesselinovitch SD, Mihailovich N (1983) Kinetics of diethylnitrosamine hepatocarcinogenesis in the infant mouse. Cancer Res 43:4253–4259

Vesselinovitch SD, Rao KVN, Mihailovich N (1979) Neoplastic response of mouse tissues during perinatal age periods and its significance in chemical carcinogenesis. JNCI Mongr 51:239–250

Vesselinovitch SD, Hacker HJ, Bannasch P (1985) Histochemical characterization of focal hepatic lesions induced by single diethylnitrosamine treatment in infant mice. Cancer Res 45:2774–2780

Ward JM (1984) Morphology of potential preneoplastic hepatocyte lesions and liver tumors in mice and a comparison with other species. In: Popp JA (ed) Mouse liver neoplasia. Hemisphere, Washington, pp 1–26

Ward JM, Ohshima M (1985) Evidence for lack of promotion of the growth of the common naturally occurring basophilic focal hepatocellular proliferative lesions in aged F344/NCr rats by phenobarbital. Carcinogenesis 6:1255–1259

Weinbren K (1984) Precancerous states in the liver. In: Carter RL (ed) Precancerous states. Oxford University Press, London, pp 254–277

Williams GM (1980) The pathogenesis of rat liver cancer caused by chemical carcinogens. Biochim Biophys Acta 605:167–189

Williams GM (1982) Phenotypic properties of preneoplastic rat liver lesions and applications to detection of carcinogens and tumor promoters. Toxicol Pathol 10:3–10

Williams GM, Watanabe K (1978) Quantitative kinetics of development of N-2-fluorenylacetamide-induced, altered hyperplastic hepatocellular foci resistant to iron accumulation and of their reversion or persistence following removal of carcinogen. JNCI 61:113–121

Williams GM, Klaiber M, Parker SE, Farber E (1976) Nature of early appearing, carcinogen-induced liver lesions resistant to iron accumulation. JNCI 57:157–165

Zerban H, Rabes HM, Bannasch P (1985) Kinetics of cell proliferation during hepatocarcinogenesis. Eur J Cancer Clin Oncol 21:1424

Carcinogenic Risk Assessment: Are Animals Good Surrogates for Man?

I. F. H. PURCHASE

Patterns of mortality in the developed world have changed substantially over the past century as we have moved to the postinfection era. Short life expectancy due primarily to infectious diseases affecting the population at an early age has changed to a much longer life expectancy due to the dramatic reduction in these infectious diseases. This change has produced an aged population suffering from chronic degenerative diseases – particularly degenerative diseases of the circulatory system (and other parts of the body) and cancer. This change in pattern has arisen as a consequence of changes in relative mortality and, hence, although degenerative diseases and cancer are far more frequent nowadays, the age-adjusted incidence of cancer has remained constant apart from changes for one or two sites. The high prevalence of chronic disease presents problems in medical care because by and large treatments are not effective and in prevention because causes operate over a long period making it difficult to distinguish the precise reasons why individuals or populations are suffering from the chronic disease. Attempts to control these diseases are putting more and more emphasis on the development of adequate preventive measures in order to avoid the suffering and cost involved in treating the terminal phase of the disease.

Rational prevention of any disease relies on an accurate assessment of the cause and magnitude of the risks which subsequently allow the introduction of suitable control measures. Epidemiological studies, reviewed in this volume by Sir Richard Doll, are crucial to the process of the accurate assessment of risks. However, problems in the conduct of epidemiological studies, particularly in the definition of adequate cohorts and the accurate assessment of exposure, and in the post hoc nature of the data collected have created the need to develop good methods of identifying carcinogens before substantial exposure of human populations occurs.

Of course these methods will also be of value in identifying more precisely the risk factors, whether natural or manmade, responsible for increased incidences of cancer. It is this role of identifying carcinogens as part of a strategy of preventive medicine that animal studies are asked to play. It is conventional to consider the data from animal studies as the best available for assessing carcinogenic risk to man because of the similarities in biology between mammals and particularly the similarity of mechanism and morphology of cancers observed in animals and those studied in man. The short life span of experimental animals provides an added bonus by reducing the latent period between chemical exposure and the development of cancer in proportion to the life span.

The environment in which the assessment of chemical carcinogenicity takes place is characterized by public concern reflected through political pressure on toxicologists to provide opinions on carcinogenic risk which stretch the data from animal experiments to their limits and unfortunately sometimes beyond. This environment within which toxicologists are working has led to confusion between the scientific component of risk assessment on the one hand, namely the assessment of hazard and the quantitative assessment of risk to exposed populations, and, on the other, the social and political judgements which properly form a component of the assessment of the acceptability of risk and the consequences of introducing control measures. Fortunately, there is an increasing awareness of the distinction between these two roles and I certainly support the view that toxicologists should concentrate on what they are trained to do, namely, to provide good scientific evaluations of toxicology and assessments of risk which will provide risk managers and society with the best and most accurate data for risk management decisions.

An analysis of the broad patterns of cancer between population groups has allowed the identification of general causes of cancer which might be considered preventable (Peto and Doll 1981). Not unexpectedly one of the major causes of cancer is seen to be cigarette smoking, but more surprisingly perhaps is the high proportion of cancer associated with diet. Only a relatively small proportion of all cancers can be considered to be due to synthetic chemicals either as a consequence of occupational exposure or adventitious exposure following environmental release of chemicals. Synthetic chemicals have been responsible for a dramatic improvement in lifestyle and life expectancy and as a consequence these chemicals are used on a very wide scale in developed countries. Over the past decade, media reports of the effects of chemicals, particularly large scale chemical accidents, have served to focus the attention of the public and governments on chemicals and their safety.

The consideration of the use of animals for assessing cancer hazard is based predominantly on the experience of testing synthetic chemicals. It might be considered that this does not adequately reflect the full range of practical uses to which animal studies may be put in the overall aim of preventing human cancer. In particular I have not addressed the contribution that animal studies have made to an assessment of the nutritional causes of cancer which has been reviewed recently by Newberne (1985). Nevertheless, some of the general principles which may be deduced from the assessment of human risk on the basis of animal carcinogenicity studies may be applicable more generally because many features of experimental design and interpretation are common to both nutritional and chemical carcinogenicity experiments.

Risk Assessment: General Principles

Risk assessment is a complex iterative process which forms part of the overall task of risk management. For ease of description and to assist in clarity of thought, risk assessment is often presented as a step-wise process (Purchase 1985). The first step is hazard identification in which animal studies and other techniques are used for identifying carcinogenic hazards. On the basis of adequate animal studies it is possible to move forward to hazard assessment in which the dose-response relationship in animals is established and the relevance of the results to man at the exposure levels likely to be experienced is assessed. Risk assessment itself integrates the information on exposure and the information on carcinogenic hazard to obtain a view on the likelihood, nature and extent of the risk in the population group exposed. Finally, the risk evaluation and the implementation of control measures involve a judgement of the acceptability of risk, including a consideration of benefits of the particular chemical, the availability of control methods and their cost. The last stage of risk management involves the implementation of controls and a review of their effectiveness and costs.

Qualitative Comparisons of Animal and Human Data

If we are to use animal studies for the purpose of hazard assessment and subsequently risk assessment, it is obviously important to define the reliability of the tests for this particular purpose. The first question that can be addressed is how well animal studies have performed in predicting human carcinogenicity in the past. One of the most reliable sets of data on the assessment of chemical carcinogenicity is the monograph series on the evaluation of carcinogenic risk of chemicals to humans produced by the International Agency for Research on Cancer. In their most recent review of 154 chemicals which have been evaluated for carcinogenicity (IARC 1982), 23 chemicals or mixtures of chemicals were listed as causally associated with cancer in humans. Of these 23 chemicals, 15 had animal carcinogenicity data which allowed a classification of "sufficient evidence of carcinogenicity" to animals. Of the remaining eight, five were classified as "limited evidence", two as "inadequate evidence" and one as not tested in animals. Poor study design, inadequate reporting or the absence of animal carcinogenicity data were the reasons why the majority of these eight chemicals had classifications which were not "sufficient evidence" in animals. The conclusion is that for all human carcinogens which have been tested adequately in animals there is sufficient evidence of carcinogenicity and for the remaining human carcinogens it is reasonable to anticipate that adequate studies will demonstrate carcinogenicity in appropriate species.

Some have been tempted to argue that because all human carcinogens have been shown to be carcinogenic in animals, the converse is true. This deduction suffers from a logical flaw (exemplified by the fact that all humans are mammals, but it is unreasonable to assume that all mammals must therefore be humans). There are practical criticisms of this conclusion based on the fact that once a chemical is known to cause cancer in man, intense efforts are made to identify the circumstances which will demonstrate carcinogenicity in animals. The reports in the 1930s and 1940s by Heuper and his colleagues described the efforts that were made in searching for an animal experimental model which would be susceptible to known human carcinogens. The criticism is confirmed by examination of the carcinogenicity data on the 23 chemicals mentioned above, where it is clear that it would not be possible to identify all of them by the use of standard carcinogenicity studies in one or two species. There is the further concern that there are hundreds of chemicals which have been shown to be carcinogenic in animals and for which the human epidemiology is negative or not adequate. It is not realistic to draw firm conclusions about the extrapolation of animal carcinogenicity data to man, particularly with respect to the false positive rate of those predictions.

If the comparative analysis of human and animal carcinogenicity data is considered inconclusive, it is an obvious step to consider carcinogenicity data from compounds studied in two species. A comparison of the carcinogenicity data on 250 chemicals in two species (Purchase 1980) has provided such a qualitative comparison of carcinogenicity. Of the 250 compounds reviewed, 38% were noncarcinogenic in both rats and mice and 44% were carcinogenic in both species. A total of 43 compounds had different results in the two species, 21 (8%) being carcinogenic in mice only, 17 (7%) in rats only and 5 (2%) having differing results from other species. From this database it is possible to calculate the sensitivity and specificity of rat studies in predicting carcinogenicity in mice and vice versa. These calculations show that the specificity (that is, the prediction of carcinogenicity) and sensitivity (that is, the prediction of noncarcinogenicity) for predicting both rat and mouse carcinogenicity studies from the other species are about 85%. It should be recognized, of course, that these predictivity figures are dramatically affected by the proportion of carcinogens in any sample of chemicals tested. If there are only 10% carcinogens in a group of chemicals tested, the predictive value for a positive result from both rat and mouse studies would be only 27%.

A comparison of the major target organs affected by the chemicals carcinogenic in both species revealed that 64% of the chemicals produced cancer at the same site (Purchase 1980).

Quantitative Comparisons of Animal and Human Data

Many aspects of the qualitative comparison of carcinogenicity are unsatisfactory, not the least of which is the fact that the data are simplified to an overall positive or negative categorization. The calculation of potency of the carcinogenic effect provides substantial additonal information

The attempts that have been made to calculate potency figures for chemical carcinogens can easily lead to the mistaken impression that potency, expressed say as the TD50 (see below), is a constant describing a characteristic of the chemical in the same way that melting point or boiling point describes a chemical characteristic. It is worth reflecting that there are at least two components involved in the expression of potency: the chemical and the host. Even within the same host the expression of potency can vary depending on tumour type, nutritional status, environmental conditions and other variables. In the same way the LD50 value describing the lethal dose can vary in the same species and is difficult to reproduce between laboratories. When considering comparisons of potency between species from the purely theoretical point of view, it would be exceedingly surprising if there were a fixed and constant ratio between the potency of carcinogenic effect in different species at different doses.

Recently, the expression of potency of chemical carcinogens has been embodied in the concept of a TD50. This is defined as the dose rate (in mg/kg body weight/day) which, if administered chronically for a standard period, would halve the probability of an animal remaining tumourless (Peto et al. 1984). This is a useful single index describing the potency of a chemical, but requires a number of statistical manipulations, including corrections for an experiment shorter than the standard period and for intercurrent mortality. Other aspects of potency including the number of organs affected and the degree of malignancy of the neoplasms are obviously not incorporated.

Attempts have been made to compare the relative potency of carcinogens in animals and man. Meselson (1975) compared the approximate total doses required to produce cancer in humans and in experimental animals. The data indicate some fairly large differences in the susceptibility of laboratory animals and man to the effects of the six carcinogens studied; for some comparisons this difference was as large as 1000-fold. A further comparison of the potencies of chemical carcinogens to animals and man was made using the slope of the dose-response curve (measured as kg · day/mg) as an indication of potency (Crouch and Wilson 1979). The ratio between the potency of chemicals in mouse and man averages about 5 : 1, with the range being from 2 : 1 to 150 : 1. Similarly the ratio of potencies for rat to man averages about 5 : 1, but varies from 1500 : 1 to 1 : 50. Attempts to make these comparisons are bedevilled by the range of potency figures that can be derived from a single species and the fact that the target organ in man and animals is frequently different. If we accept the enormous importance of accurate carcinogenic risk assessment only the most enthusiastic would take this comparative data as a strong indication of a good correlation in potency between species. The number of human carcinogens for which there is adequate data make comparison with animal data somewhat constrained.

As for qualitative comparisons, the next obvious step was to examine the data for chemicals which were carcinogenic in two species to see if the potency estimates were similar. I have already commented on the fact that potency estimates for chemical carcinogens are likely to be moderated by biological variables including the species and strain used, the route of administration and the environmental conditions under which the animals are kept. The large series of carcinogenicity studies carried out under the auspices of the National Cancer Institute (NCI) or National Toxicology Program (NTP) in the USA provide an ideal opportunity for comparisons of carcinogenic potency. In these experiments many of the confounding factors are controlled by careful attention to protocol and by the selection of the same strain and species and the use of the same batch of chemical for carcinogenicity tests. Several studies have been carried out of the quantitative relationship between carcinogenicity in rats and mice. In one of these studies (Crouch 1983), the data from the carcinogenicity testing of 187 chemicals in rats and mice in the NCI bioassay series were compared. A comparison of the carcinogenic potency of 78 chemicals in the $B6C3F_1$ mouse and in the F344 rat revealed that in general there was a correlation between the carcinogenic potency in these two species. The method of computation of potency (as a function of the integrated life time dose and tumour incidence) allowed the calculation of confidence limits for the potency estimates. As a consequence it was possible to calculate the standard deviation about the correlation, producing a value of 0.66. This implied that the uncertainties in extrapolating between rats and mice were larger than was generally acknowledged, as the standard deviation of the comparison was a factor of about 4.5. Using this technique it was also possible to compare chemicals for which results were positive in one species but negative in the other. Such a comparison showed no obvious exceptions to the general rule deduced from chemicals carcinogenic in both species. However, one further important conclusion was that the confidence intervals – calculated solely on the basis of group size and the binomial distribution – do not explain the variance between species. Hence the differences in potency, including the negative results, are not the consequence of statistical limitations of the study but rather demonstrate a real difference in potency between the species. Finally the authors were unable to find evidence of any obvious exceptional cases to the general relationship of potency between the two species.

Two years later, Bernstein and his colleagues (1986) revealed a problem when using the NCI/NTP data for such comparisons. They examined the data from 186 NCI carcinogenicity experiments and were able to show that there was a very strong correlation between the maximum doses used in rats and mice ($r^2 = 0.82$, on a logarithmic scale). The range of carcinogenic potencies which can be obtained from a "standard" NCI/NTP protocol is restricted to about 30-fold, largely because of the limited range of increases in tumour incidence that can be observed in such a study. As the maximum doses used in the series of experiments vary over many orders of magnitude, it necessarily follows that the potency must be correlated between the two species when derived from this data set. The conclusion that one can draw on the basis of Bernstein's observation is that an important and unexpected confounding effect has been observed which prevents us from drawing firm conclusions about whether or not there is a good potency correlation between rats and mice based on the NCI/NTP data.

Correlations between biological data derived from animal experiments have provided other unexpected results. One such comparison has described the close correlation between acute toxicity and carcinogenic potency (Zeise et al. 1984). Using data from the same series of experiments as those studied by Crouch (1983) and data available in the literature on acute toxicity, it was found that there is a correlation between the carcinogenic potency computed from the NCI studies and the LD50 value derived from acute toxicity studies. This comparison looks statistically sensible, but it is an affront to toxicologists who view the mechanisms of acute toxicity as substantially different from those in chronic toxicity. Nevertheless, Zeise proceeds to describe a method of using acute toxicity as a predictor of carcinogenicity with a scheme assessing carcinogenicity based on acute toxicity as the first step. In view of the observations made by Bernstein, it may well be possible to provide an explanation for the improbable association between acute toxicity and carcinogenicity. There is a reasonably constant relationship between the maximum tolerated dose in a long-term carcinogenicity experiment and the LD50 of the chemical under test; indeed the maximum dose and other doses are sometimes set as a fraction of the LD50. Bernstein has shown a strong relationship between the maximum tolerated doses in different species and how this affects the assessment of potency. Thus, the problems confronting us in attempts to compare carcinogenicity between species are also faced by those comparing numerical indices of acute toxicity with carcinogenic potency.

The belief that data from animal carcinogenicity studies is directly and immediately relevant to human cancer hazard assessment creates a further practical problem. The current practice in the design of animal carcinogenicity studies is to test chemicals under fairly rigorous conditions in order to avoid the pitfall of false negative results. The consequence is that the maximum dose selected is frequently very much larger than that experienced by human populations exposed to the chemical concerned and for practical purposes the group sizes of such animal experiments are in the range of 50–100 animals per group. Results from these data are extrapolated to man assuming that the most sensitive result from the most sensitive species is the appropriate result to use for extrapolation to man and that there is a simple direct quantitative correlation between these results and the expected effect in man. The consequence of this philosophy is to present to the epidemiologist the hypothesis that the chemical concerned will produce cancer in an exposed population at a particular very low incidence. The epidemiologist in testing this hypothesis will be dealing with low relative risks and a low number of expected tumours because of the usual small cohort size and the fact that most of the cohort is still alive. This combination presents formidable problems to the epidemiologist in that in order to have a reasonable chance of disproving the hypothesis an enormous cohort study must be carried out to provide suitable statistical power. The result of this sequence of events is that we find ourselves in the curious situation of using data from epidemiological studies, which is ultimately the most useful in the assessment of carcinogenic risk, to try to disprove a hypothesis which is based on a sequence of untestable assumptions.

Quantitative Extrapolation from Animal Data

Toxicologists traditionally use safety factors to define a dose below the no-observed-effect level which is unlikely to cause harm to a population exposed to the chemical. This safety factor, an empirical figure of about 100, is often rationalized as providing a 10-fold safety factor for interspecies differences and a 10-fold factor for variations in susceptibility within the human population. Over the years the safety factor approach has been shown to work well for acute toxicity, but for a number of reasons a more sophisticated approach was deemed desirable for the extrapolation of carcinogenicity data. In principle, a better quantitative method of extrapolation should improve quantitative risk assessment. A variety of mathematical models has been developed whose purpose is to calculate the expected risk at doses far below those in the observed range. These mathematical techniques are based on a variety of assumptions which it is not important to develop here; however, there are often a variety of unstated assumptions which are very important in an assessment of the utility of these models. These assumptions include: (a) the animal data are qualitatively and quantitatively reliable for extrapolation to man; (b) the dose-response relationship at low doses is linear; (c) some of the principles on which the mathematical models are developed are loosely compatible with current concepts of the multistage processes involved in carcinogenesis.

The use of quantitative extrapolation for regulatory purposes has been pioneered by the Cancer Assessment Group of the Environmental Protection Agency (EPA), USA (Anderson 1985). The EPA has selected the multistage model to compute a q value which represents the maximum likelihood estimate of the slope of the dose-response relationship. More frequently the EPA prefers to use the q^* value which is the 95% upper confidence limit of the slope of the dose-response relationship. This technique has the benefit of simplifying the calculation of risk at any given dose because the dose-response relationship is linearized. Many toxicologists view this practice with considerable scepticism because the technique aims to be conservative, it is unverifiable, and the estimates of risk vary more as a consequence of the selection of the model than of the biological data on which the risk assessment is based.

Against this background of apparent conflict between statisticians and toxicologists, it is worth asking whether the use of a sophisticated mathematical model is in

Table 1. Comparison of carcinogenic potency indices

Compounds	(a) Slope $(mg/kg/day)^{-1}$	(b) Dose for 10^{-6} risk	(c) TD50 (mg)	(c/b)
Acrylonitrile	0.24	4.17×10^{-5}	5.31	1.27×10^{5}
Aflatoxin B1	2900	3.45×10^{-9}	0.0009	2.6×10^{5}
Aldrin	11.4	8.77×10^{-7}	0.740	8.43×10^{5}
Arsenic	15			
B[a]P	11.5	8.69×10^{-7}	1.86	2.13×10^{6}
Benzene	2.9×10^{-2}	3.45×10^{-4}	77	2.2×10^{5}
Benzidene	234	4.27×10^{-8}	2	4.68×10^{7}
Carbon tetrachloride	1.30×10^{-1}	7.69×10^{-5}	0.88	1.14×10^{4}
Chlordane	1.61	6.2×10^{-6}	1.45	2.33×10^{5}
Chlorinated ethanes				
1,2-Dichloroethane	6.9×10^{-2}	1.4×10^{-4}	5.49	3.9×10^{4}
Hexachloroethane	1.42×10^{-2}	7.0×10^{-4}	319	4.5×10^{5}
1,1,2,2-Tetrachloroethane	0.20	5.0×10^{-5}	35.4	7.08×10^{5}
1,1,2-Trichloroethane	5.73×10^{-2}	1.74×10^{-4}	47.6	2.7×10^{5}
Chloroform	7×10^{-2}	1.42×10^{-4}	48	3.36×10^{5}
DDT	0.34	2.9×10^{-5}	4.55	1.54×10^{5}
Dichlorobenzidine	1.69	6.1×10^{-6}	18.3	3.00×10^{6}
1,1-Dichloroethylene (vinylidene chloride)	1.47×10^{-1}	6.8×10^{-5}	23.6	3.47×10^{5}
Dieldrin	30.4	3.29×10^{-7}	0.567	1.72×10^{6}
2,4-Dinitrotoluene	0.31	3.22×10^{-5}	9.35	3.0×10^{5}
Bis(2-chloroethyl)ether	1.14	8.77×10^{-6}	8.19	9.33×10^{5}
Bis(chloromethyl)ether	9300	1.07×10^{-9}	0.00357	3.32×10^{6}
Ethylene dibromide (EDB)	41	2.43×10^{-7}	1.1	4.51×10^{6}
Heptachlor	3.37	3.00×10^{-6}	1.09	3.67×10^{5}
Hexachlorobenzene	1.67	6.0×10^{-6}	5.48	9.15×10^{5}
Hexachlorobutadiene	7.75×10^{-2}	1.29×10^{-4}	50.5	3.91×10^{5}
Hexachlorocyclohexane				
Alpha isomer	11.12	8.9×10^{-7}	11.2	1.2×10^{7}
Beta isomer	1.84	5.4×10^{-6}	17.7	3.26×10^{6}
Gamma isomer	1.33	7.51×10^{-6}	17.7	2.35×10^{6}
Nitrosamines				
Dimethylnitrosamine	25.9	3.86×10^{-7}	0.113	2.89×10^{5}
Diethylnitrosamine	43.5	2.30×10^{-7}	0.00787	3.4×10^{4}
Dibutylnitrosamine	5.43	1.84×10^{-6}	0.686	3.72×10^{5}
N-nitrosopyrrolidine	2.13	4.69×10^{-6}	2.51	5.35×10^{5}
N-nitroso-N-methylurea	302.6	3.3×10^{-8}	3.0	9.07×10^{7}
N-nitroso-diphenylamine	4.92×10^{-3}	2.03×10^{-3}	201	10.0×10^{4}
Phenols				
2,4,6-Trichlorophenol	1.99×10^{-2}	5.02×10^{-4}	68	1.35×10^{5}
Tetrachlorodibenzo-p-dioxin (TCDD)	1.56×10^{-5}	6.4×10^{-11}	0.000006	9.36×10^{4}

Table 1 (continued)

Compounds	(a) Slope $(mg/kg/day)^{-1}$	(b) Dose for 10^{-6} risk	(c) TD50 (mg)	(c/b)
Tetrachloroethylene	6.0×10^{-2}	1.66×10^{-4}	75.6	4.54×10^{5}
Trichloroethylene	1.2×10^{-2}	8.3×10^{-9}	16.9	2.03×10^{4}
Vinyl chloride	1.75×10^{-2}	5.7×10^{-4}	0.761	1.33×10^{3}

(a) Figure calculated by EPA
(b) Calculated from (a)
(c) The lowest value for the chemical in Gold et al. (1984)

fact superior to the use of a safety factor. This problem has been addressed by the calculation of a "virtually safe dose" by using a safety factor of 5000 and applying it to the lowest effective dose from animal carcinogenicity studies (Hoel 1985). Doses were calculated in this way for 15 compounds to establish whether reliable estimates of low-dose risk were produced. Using these calculated doses, the carcinogenic risk was computed using the upper confidence limit of the multistage model. Had the two methods of calculation agreed, a constant would be expected. However, the result was that a wide range of risks was observed and it was concluded that safety factors had no place to play in the assessment of carcinogenic risk at low doses. Some may feel that this conclusion was based on an unwise decision to use a mathematical model, which itself is suspect, in order to derive data to invalidate an alternative method of computing risk at low dose.

This issue leads directly to the question of the relationship between observations in the experimental range and those at lower doses. The recent development of the concept of the TD50 allows a comparison between effects in the experimental range and those at much lower doses. As the mathematical models used assume linearity of the dose-response relationship, it is possible to calculate the dose likely to produce a 50% incidence of tumours ($q \times 5 \times 10^{-1}$) and the dose to produce a 10^{-6} risk ($q \times 10^{-6}$). The relationship between these two doses is a constant, namely, 5×10^{-5}. This theoretical relationship is confirmed by comparing the two values for 38 carcinogens (Table 1). For 34 of these the ratio is between 10^4 and 10^6. It has recently been demonstrated that TD50 values can be estimated quite adequately using summary incidence date rather than the full life table data originally described for its estimation (Gold et al. 1986). It may turn out that a much easier method of calculating the "virtually safe dose" computed to produce a risk of 10^{-6} is to divide the TD50 by 5×10^5.

Design, Interpretation and Usefulness of Animal Studies

The design of any toxicological study should be determined by the hypothesis to be tested and the use to which the results are to be put. There are rarely absolute criteria available which have been tested by experiment, particularly when designing carcinogenicity studies. The protocols for carcinogenicity studies have been refined over the past two decades and there is now general agreement about many features of carcinogenicity study design which are published in guidelines by national and

Table 2. Incidence of most frequent neoplasms in rats, mice[a] and humans[b]

F344 Rats		B6C3F1 Mice		H. sapiens		
Site	%	Site	%	ICD no.	Site	%
Males						
Testes	82.3	Liver	24.6	162	Trachea, bronchus and lung	7.6
Leukaemia/lymphoma	19.9	Lung/bronchi/trachea	13.7	173	Skin	3.1
Pituitary	14.7	Leukaemia/lymphoma	10.3	185	Prostate	2.5
Adrenal	12.4	Skin	3.1	151	Stomach	2.0
Thyroid	8.2	Circulatory system	2.9	153	Colon	1.9
Skin	7.8	Adrenal	1.4	188	Bladder	1.9
Pancreas	3.9	Thyroid	1.0	154	Rectum	1.5
Lung/bronchi/trachea	3.0	Testes	0.4	204–208	Leukaemia	0.62
Preputial gland	2.4			186	Testes	0.25
Liver	2.2			155	Liver	0.16
Females						
Pituitary	34.9	Leukaemia/lymphoma	20.6	174	Breast	5.8
Mammary gland	20.9	Lung/bronchi/trachea	5.2	173	Skin	2.7
Uterus	17.0	Liver	4.7	162	Trachea, bronchus and lung	2.5
Leukaemia/lymphoma	13.4	Pituitary	3.6	153	Colon	2.2
Thyroid	6.8	Circulatory system	2.4	151	Stomach	1.3
Adrenal	5.2	Skin	1.7	154	Rectum	1.2
Skin	3.2	Thyroid	1.7	183	Ovary	1.2
Lung/bronchi/trachea	1.9	Uterus	1.6	180	Cervix	1.1
Liver	1.9	Mammary gland	1.3	204–208	Leukaemia	0.48
Preputial gland	1.8			194	Pituitary	0.01

[a] Data from Chu et al. (1981)

[b] Data calculated by GM Paddle using the percentage of persons registered as cancer patients and assuming a life span of 70 years (based on registrations in England and Wales, 1982)

international organizations. These protocols have been developed from the distilled wisdom of a group of toxicologists; it is rare to have justification for particular details in the protocol on the basis of systematic experiment and comparison of the results with the final extrapolation for which the results will be used. In this respect carcinogenicity studies differ substantially from chemical analytical techniques which are thoroughly tested before their introduction. The main reason for this difference is the expense of investigating aspects of carcinogenicity protocols. The criteria which are now used seem to have developed on the basis of avoiding previous mistakes, avoiding obvious confounding factors and to maximize the likelihood of obtaining a positive outcome. It is rare to see an analysis of detailed components of the protocol of long-term carcinogenicity studies for their impact on the consequent use of the data for hazard assessment.

The criteria which are considered in the design of a long-term carcinogenicity study are numerous, covering both the external environment, the experimental manipulations and the way observations are made. Most guidelines provide information on the species to be selected and usually the principle is that the species used should be selected on the basis of similarities in metabolism between that species and man. In practice the vast majority of carcinogenicity studies are carried out on rats and mice, in spite of the fact that there is a great body of knowledge about differences in metabolism and other aspects of the carcinogenic process between rodents and man. One obvious difference is longevity and it is perhaps lucky that latency appears to be related to longevity. Another major difference is the neoplasms observed in untreated groups. Neoplasms with the highest incidence in rats and mice are not only different from those observed in man (Table 2), but also occur at very much higher incidence rates. How should we deal with such massive differences in incidence rates? At the moment the only answer to that question is the application of suitable statistical significance techniques to correct for high background incidences of cancer.

Another important feature in the protocol of animal studies is the diagnostic criteria used by the pathologist in judging whether a neoplasm is benign or malignant. This difficulty is usually overcome by relying on the consensus of opinion of a team of pathologists. There is a recent example which illustrates the difficulties confronting the pathologist in this area. Up until 1981 the incidence of mononuclear cell leukaemia in NTP studies rarely exceeded 20% in female rats and 40% in male rats. From the middle of 1982 the incidence increased substantially so that the mean values were 25% for female rats and 49% for male rats in 1983. This change in the incidence of mononuclear cell leukaemia in control animals appears to have originated from a change in diagnostic criteria following a conference of pathologists in 1982 (Rao, personal communication) although no other changes as large as those observed for leukaemia have been reported. This is confirmed in a broader range of studies by the observation that the major sources of variability in historical control rates are calendar year and laboratory (Haseman 1984). The question that remains to be answered is whether these changes in diagnostic criteria make the animal experiments more useful or less useful for their primary purpose of assessing human carcinogenic risk.

There is frequently an argument that the results from certain types of outcome from carcinogenicity studies are less reliable in predicting human cancer risk than are the majority of results. For example, it is argued that tumours which occur at high and variable incidence in experimental animals, such as lung and liver tumours in mice, are less valuable in predicting human cancer than are changes in incidence of other tumours. Those who disagree with this argument often claim that the danger of false negative results should lead us to rely on all data from animal carcinogenicity studies. Both of these arguments appear somewhat superficial and more details of mechanistic differences and similarities should help in resolving the issue. There are a number of examples where there are clear mechanistic reasons why data from animal studies should carry less weight. One example is that of liver cancer. There is generally a much higher incidence in rodents, particularly mice, than in man. It is known that environmental factors such as dietary intake can modulate the tumour incidence suggesting that the biology of rodent liver cancer may be substantially different from that in man. Studies of cellular development in liver have demonstrated that mitosis and cytokinesis do not necessarily follow consecutively with the result that in some species polyploidy and binuclearity is common, whilst in others it is rare. Amongst rodents polyploidy is common in rats, mice and hamsters, but not in guinea pigs. In aged mice the average ploidy of liver cells may be $16n$. In contrast polyploidy does not occur to any extent in primates although some $2 \times 2n$ cells have been reported in aged humans. These differences in cell development in rodent liver may well explain the different responses of rodent liver to xenobiotics.

There are other examples of clear differences in the biology of cancer between rodents and man. Rat mammary carcinomata are prolactin sensitive and higher incidences are seen in animals with prolactin-secreting pituitary adenomas. The sensitivity of mammary carcinomas in rats to the effects of oestrogens differs from that in man where oestrogens may be used in the treatment of some forms of mammary cancer. It seems that any chemical which will alter the hormone levels, particularly at high doses, may modulate the incidence of mammary carcinoma in rats in a way which is not likely to occur in man, especially at low doses.

A further set of examples, all of which relate to local tissue damage, seem to provide data which are inappropriate for human risk assessment. Early work on bladder carcinoma which involved the implantation of cholesterol and glass beads has shown unequivocally that the presence of solid material in the rodent bladder results in a high incidence of bladder carcinoma. The administration of chemicals, such as ethylene glycol, which result in extensive precipitation of stones in the bladder, can produce a high incidence of bladder carcinoma. In the elegant work of Weil (1965), it was shown that the transplantation of bladder stones from ethylene glycol-treated animals to control animals resulted in the appearance of bladder cancer in the control animals, whilst none appeared in the ethylene glycol-treated animals. Clearly the presence of bladder stones in rodents is a confounding factor and must be taken into account in assessing the carcinogenicity of chemicals. Similar effects are created by repeated damage to the skin which has been shown to increase the incidence of papilloma and carcinoma of the skin particularly in animals which have been initiated with a single dose of a carcinogen (Argyliss and Slaga 1981). Indeed the application to the skin of irritant chemicals, such as sodium hydroxide or hydrochloric acid, results in the induction of squamous neoplasms in mice (Navat 1925). It has been recognized for some years that repeated subcutaneous injection of chemicals can result in the induction of local sarcomas. The work of Grasso and Goldberg (1966) showed that this may be an osmotic effect as some chemicals which cause cancer after subcutaneous administration of an hypertonic solution failed to do so when the same amount was given in a more dilute solution. In addition chemicals, such as glucose, in hypertonic solution were capable of inducing subcutaneous sarcomas in rats.

These latter examples show specific cases where there is a clear link between the design of a long-term carcinogenicity study, its interpretation and subsequently the utility of those results in the assessment of human risk. It is generally agreed that glass beads should not be considered carcinogenic on the basis of the results from implantation in the bladder. It does not seem likely that sodium hydroxide or glucose should be considered as representing a carcinogenic risk on the basis of the skin painting and subcutaneous injection experiments described above. These examples make it quite clear that there is no general rule which makes all results from animal carcinogenicity studies immediately applicable to man. In every case when this extrapolation is being attempted, careful thought must be given to the mechanisms of induction in animals and their similarity to the human situation.

Conservatism in Risk Assessment

There is no doubt that there are a large number of uncertainties in the process of carcinogenic risk assessment based on animal data. These uncertainties present the toxicologist with the opportunity of choosing the assumptions which should be used in the risk assessment process. The extensive social and political pressures, presumably derived from the public fear of cancer and the belief that it is preventable, have lead to the view that all assumptions used during the risk assessment process must be "conservative". In this context conservative means that the assumption is chosen which maximizes the magnitude of risk assessed. For example, the quantitative approaches used by the EPA appear to be selected on the basis of maximizing the risk in order to determine the "upper bound" of the risk (Anderson 1985).

It is possible to use conservative assumptions in the process of risk assessment at a number of different levels. These may include: (a) the selection of the most potent result from animal carcinogenicity studies whilst ignoring all other results, including negative results; (b) utilizing data from experiments in which the maximum dose has clearly compromised the response of the animal; (c) combining benign and malignant neoplasms in the assessment of rodent carcinogenesis which will overestimate the risk in man because most benign neoplasms would not be diagnosable; (d) assuming a linear nonthreshold dose-response relationship even for nongenotoxic carcinogens; (e) selecting a one-hit or a linearized multistage model for low-dose risk assessment (this may have a profound impact on the assessment of risk; a one-hit linearized model would show a reduction of 100 in the risk if the dose was reduced by 100, whereas a similar reduction in dose would provide a reduction in risk of 10^4 for a two-hit model); (f) the use of the upper confidence limit rather than the maximum likelihood estimate; and (g) the computation of dose on the basis of surface area rather than weight, which is about 10 times more conservative – data from Crouch (1983) do not indicate that surface area is more accurate in converting doses between species than simple weight extrapolation.

Using a sequence of conservative assumptions can create wide differences in risk assessment which are not immediately apparent. If each of the six steps identified above was more conservative than the real situation by a factor of 5, the overall assessment would be in error by a factor of 15625 (5^6). The information given to risk managers by using these conservative assessment procedures is biased in a way which is prejudged by the toxicologist. This may be particularly important where the risk manager must balance the risks and benefits associated with two different strategies, one of which involves carcinogenicity and the other not. Asymmetries in conservatism in this situation can produce misallocations of control efforts (Nichols and Zeckhauser 1985).

Conclusion

This paper has attempted to address the question of whether animals are good surrogates for man in carcinogenic risk assessment. Risk assessment is the scientific component of the overall risk management of carcinogens and therefore deliberate over- or underestimation of risk during the scientific phase of risk management is in no-one's interest. There is no doubt that human carcinogens can be shown to be carcinogenic in animals. Equally there is strong evidence to support the view that no simple screening strategy using standard animal carcinogenicity studies will be 100% accurate in predicting carcinogenictiy and noncarcinogenicity. In particular there are a variety of mechanistic data which suggest that certain responses in experimental animals (for example, local sarcoma after repeated subcutaneous injection and bladder cancer after bladder stone formation) are simply not applicable to the human situation. Attempts so far to provide empirical evidence that quantitative data from animal carcinogenicity studies are useful in predicting human risk have been thwarted by the small number of human carcinogens identified and by the presence of confounding factors within the experimental data available.

The process of risk assessment has many steps and is complex. At each step a number of assumptions have to be made in order to proceed to the following step. In light of the uncertainty about the mechanisms of chemical carcinogenesis, it is easy to provide conservative assumptions at each stage in the risk assessment process. It has become clear that the product of multiple conservative assumptions is likely to provide unrealistic estimates of risk. When there is asymmetry in the conservatism used in the risk assessment process, particularly, say, between that for a carcinogenic risk and a noncarcinogenic risk, there is likely to be misallocation of resources for controlling the risks. Under these circumstances it can hardly be considered that animals are acting as good surrogates for man. However, if risk assessment takes into account knowledge of mechanisms of action and attempts to provide the most accurate assessment of risk, with an indication of the margins of error, data from animal carcinogenicity studies will prove increasingly useful in predicting human carcinogenic risk. When careful attention is paid to the detailed scientific issues at every stage of risk assessment, animals can be seen as adequate surrogates for man in the sense that they allow for the implementation of appropriate control measures which will protect populations from unacceptable risks of cancer.

References

Anderson EL (1985) Quantitative approaches in use in the United States to assess cancer risk. In: Vouk VB, Butler GC, Hoel DG, Peakall DB (eds) Methods for estimating risk of chemical injury: human and non-human biota and ecosystems. Wiley, Chichester, pp 405–436

Argyliss TS, Slaga TJ (1981) Promotion of carcinomas by repeated abrasion in initiated skin of mice. Cancer Res 41:5193–5195

Bernstien L, Gold LS, Ames BN, Pike MC, Hoel DG (1985) Some tautologous aspects of the comparison of carcinogenic potency in rats and mice. Fundam Appl Toxicol 5:79–86

Chu KC, Cueto C, Ward JM (1981) Factors in the evaluation of 200 National Cancer Institute carcinogen bioassays. J Toxicol Environ Health 8:251

Crouch E, Wilson R (1979) Interspecies comparison of carcinogenic potency. J Toxicol Environ Health 5:1095–1118

Crouch EAC (1983) Uncertainties in interspecies extrapolations of carcinogenicity. Environ Health Perspect 50:321–327

EPA (1985) Mutagenicity and carcinogenicity assessment of 1,3-butadiene. Final report. EPA/600/8-85 004F Office of Health, Environmental Assessment, United States Environmental Protection Agency, Washington DC 20460

Gold LS, Sawyer CB, Magaw R, Backman GM, de Veciana M, Levinson R, Hooper NK, Havender WR, Bernstein L, Peto R, Pike MC, Ames BN (1984) A carcinogenic potency database of the standardized results of animal bioassays. Environ Health Perspect 58:9–319

Gold LS, Bernstein L, Kaldor J, Backman G, Hoel D (1986) An empirical comparison of methods used to estimate carcinogenic potency in long-term animal bioassays: lifetable vs summary incidence date. Fundam Appl Toxicol 6:263–269

Grasso P, Golberg L (1966) Subcutaneous sarcoma as an index of carcinogenic potency. Fd Cosmet Toxicol 4:297–320

Haseman JK (1984) Statistical issues in the design analysis and interpretation of animal carcinogenicity studies. Environ Health Perspect 58:385–392

Hoel DG (1985) Mathematical dose-response models and their application to risk estimation. In: Vouk VB, Butler GC, Hoel DG, Peakall DB (eds) Methods for estimating risk of chemical injury: human and nonhuman biota and ecosystems. Wiley, Chichester, pp 347–360

IARC (1982) Monographs on the evaluation of the carcinogenic risk of chemicals to humans, supplement 4. International Agency for Research on Cancer, Lyon

Meselson MS (1975) Contemporary test control practices and prospects. The report of the executive committee, NAS, Washington, DC, p 75

Navat JK (1925) Experimental production of malignant growth by simple chemicals. J Cancer Res 9:135–147

Newberne P (1985) The influence of nutrition, immunologic status and other factors on the development of cancer. In: Clayson DB, Krewski D, Munro I (eds) Toxicological risk assessment. CRC Press, Boca Raton, pp 43–88

Nichols AL, Zeckhauser RJ (1985) The dangers of caution: conservatism in assessment and the mismanagement of risk. Discussion paper series, John F Kennedy School of Government, Harvard University

Peto R, Doll R (1981) Quantitative estimates of avoidable risks in cancer in United States today. JNCI 66:1191–1308

Peto R, Pike MC, Bernstein L, Gold LS, Ames BN (1984) The Td50; a proposed general convention for the numerical description of the carcinogenic potency of chemicals in chronic-exposure animal experiments. Environ Health Perspect 58:1–8

Purchase IFH (1980) Inter-species comparisons of carcinogenicity. Br J Cancer 41:454–468

Purchase IFH (1985) Carcinogenic risk assessment: a toxicologist's view. Banbury Rep (Risk quantitation and regulatory policy) 19:175–186

Weil CS (1965) Urinary bladder response to diethylene glycol: calculi and tumours following repeated feeding and implants. Arch Environ Health 11:569–581

Zeise L, Wilson R, Crouch E (1984) Use of acute toxicity to estimate carcinogenic risk. Risk Analysis 4:187–199

Summary of Discussion: Session 2

R. Bass

The starting point for all discussions was the statement that the ill-considered move from some "positive" experimental data to classification of a chemical substance as "human carcinogen" cannot be recommended. Some of the many reasons offered to support this cautious statement are outlined below.

Practicability

In recent years the number of substances that have turned out to be "carcinogenic" in long-term studies in animals – so-called bioassays – has increased steadily (the term bioassay is often used to describe a long-term animal study performed to assess "carcinogenicity." Experimental conditions and necessary preliminary studies have been laid down, for example, by the USA-NTP program, but they are subject to change). Over time one would expect more substances to carry such a label than not. It is questionable, however, whether all of these compounds should also be classified as human carcinogens. Although the validity of bioassay data is not in doubt, therefore, additional criteria need to be developed to allow regulation of those chemical substances which exert a strong carcinogenic influence.

Scientific Development

There are only a very few exceptions to the rule that "all human carcinogens are animal carcinogens." Scientific understanding has advanced to explain such exceptions. The inverse, i.e., "all animal carcinogens are human carcinogens," was also claimed to be true and for a long time was taken for granted. However, many problems became evident in the extrapolation of bioassay data to the carcinogenic risk of chemicals in man more recently. Now that the general necessity of considering peculiarities of exposure, pharmacokinetics, and possible mechanisms of action has been recognized for some time, these aspects will have to be concentrated on in the future by seeking special information tailored to the properties of the substance investigated. The experimental burden will either be on establishing dose-response relationships, on revealing pharmacokinetic peculiarities, on establishing comparable and accessible endpoints – apart from tumors – in the experimental model system and in man, or in a combination of several of these. As a rule, all data available for the compound to be judged have to be considered, but their use for risk assessment should be based on their relevance for man. The number and type of useful data that can be obtained is constantly increasing.

Validation of Test Systems

In spite of the difficulties of the extrapolation of animal data to man, bioassays still form the heart of the classification of chemicals as carcinogens. Scientific recognition of validation criteria for bioassay data has focused on across-species differences, reproducibility, and (in)congruence with results from short-term tests and from human studies. However, no clear-cut structure has developed so far that could reliably and understandably be employed in those cases where the experiments in animals may not adequately reflect the situation in man. Unless such structures are developed there will be no other choice than to regulate and classify such compounds by extrapolation from bioassay data. Assessment of validity of short-term tests among single test systems, among themselves, and in comparison with data from other study types has been recognized as an absolute prerequisite before plugging them into test schemes for risk assessment.

Apparent Problems of Today's Classification Schemes

Undoubtedly the classification scheme of IARC (a subdivision of the WHO) has formed an indispensable basis for national and international regulation and handling of carcinogenic risk, whenever a compound has been dealt with by this agency. However, we must not forget that IARC's liaison with regulation is to supply administrators with a critical scientific assembly of available data and assessment of these data according to their own rules.

Transposition of IARC's assessment for regulatory needs has to incorporate, for instance, actual or past exposure data in order to interprete the significance of a carcinogenic potential disclosed in bioassays. Interpretation for regulation has to reach beyond a "yes/no" classification of toxic potentials and one has to lay down rules for occupational or other exposure/uses. Possible decisions span from total prohibition through restrictions of use(s) (e.g., MAK values in the Federal Republic of Germany), or replacement by other substances, to no regulatory restriction.

From this starting point of the discussion on how to transfer experimental data into classification of chemicals, a large number of more general and specific questions arose. For many of them there is no answer available today; for some of them not even an unarguable opinion can be obtained. In summarizing they can be grouped as in the next section.

From Experimental Results to Risk Assessment for Man

Definitions. It was recognized that the same terms in the past have been used with different meanings. "Risk" and "hazard" are still employed in opposing senses (e.g., by WHO and in Anglo-saxon countries) regarding the description of qualitative (potential) and quantitative (actual occurring) ability (potency) to induce carcinogenic effects. The terms "risk" and "hazard" should either not be employed to differentiate between qualitative and quantitative descriptions of the chances for man to develop cancer, or should be employed according to WHO usage. WHO (1978) Principles and methods for evaluating the toxicity of chemicals. Environ Health Criteria 6(1): 19–20.

Using hepatocellular events as an example, the importance of correct terminology was stressed. Terms like preneoplastic/neoplastic, qualitative or quantitative regression of lesions/persistence, benign/malignant, foci/nodules/tumor/carcinoma should be employed by strictly adhering to the morphological and histological nomenclature introduced by pathologists. Difficulties concerning the use of these terms, however, arise when judgment (diagnosis) is to be made while the fate of the lesions observed is experimentally unknown, because the final lesion is not yet available or cannot be made available (short-term tests). Prediction then solely relies on experience and opinion. Although one might expect, for instance, that, given enough time, "hepatic nodules" will progress to tumors, the actual occurrence or frequency of tumors cannot be assessed from nodules alone. Apparently it is also possible that some types of such "nodules" will regress and not give rise to carcinomas. When the nodules persist, however, for some weeks after withdrawal of the chemical in "stop experiments," this appears to be a reliable indicator of carcinogenic potential of the compound tested.

Another important aspect was the discussion of whether it can be considered acceptable to lump together data on "nodules" and "carcinoma" in order to establish a dose-response. Strong objections were raised against such policy, which has frequently been applied during risk assessment in the past.

Similarly, difficulties must arise when pathologists change their view in interpreting lesions, as has happened, e.g., with some hepatocellular lesions which are no longer classified as carcinoma. Historical comparisons have to be adjusted accordingly, which will often be impossible to perform.

Difficulties must also be expected when a substance is classified as a "weak" or "strong" mutagen. Plain description of results is to be preferred.

Short-Term Tests. The conditions of culture and the inverse relationship between drug metabolizing capabilities (total and vs time) and growth potential (total or lifespan) was accepted as one experimental challenge of in vitro short-term testing of today; thus rendering such tests difficult to use in a routine manner. Although cocultivation experiments with metabolically competent (liver) cells still pose problems, they may better mimic in vivo conditions (e.g., cell–cell interaction) by quite a degree and may help to overcome the deficiencies encountered by using a single cell type.

In vivo short-term tests have been proposed as *indirect* information or evidence on the possible occurrence of substance-related tumors. With the exception of clofibrate, its analogues, and other peroxisome proliferation inducers, apparently all experimental liver carcinogens hitherto investigated are also able to induce focal lesions. Assumption of the inverse relationship (all substances inducing focal liver lesions will eventually lead to liver tumors) would lead to the proposal that the occurrence of foci supplies *direct* evidence for the ultimate occurrence of tumors. When assuming such a sequence of events, some pitfalls, however, still exist. These concern, for instance, the use of a different species (e.g., mice instead of rats), or a very rapid progression of tumor development where foci as a transitional stage may not have been grasped.

To relate such events to the possible occurrence of hepatocellular tumors in man, other problems have yet to be considered. Since differences in organ-specificity have to be expected, it is interesting to note that known human liver carcinogens experimentally lead to foci development. Other organs (experience mainly relying on kidney and pancreas) exhibit focal lesions less frequently, and these are moreover hard to diagnose.

From Experimental Results to Risk Assessment for Man. During the discussion a clear warning was expressed that it is unwise to label substances for positive carcinogenicity too early (regulatory needs may and indeed have overruled this). To allow necessary labeling early, extrapolation from qualitative evaluation should only be employed for substances exhibiting a "strong" carcinogenic potential. Interpretation of action as "weak" or "unclear" carcinogenic potential should lead to attempts for quantification of effects first. Quantification attempts can and should employ the whole variety of supportive test systems available, from in vitro and in vivo short-term tests to biological dosimetry. Thus the specific needs for individual substances to allow extrapolation from experimental systems to man (via pharmacokinetic, metabolic, and biochemical investigations, including dose-response relationship studies on in vivo and in vitro helper-targets, or via studies on the mechanism of action) can best be accommodated.

Several weak spots were stressed in attempts to quantify effects most of them related to the shape of dose-response curves, extent of repair at low doses, and knowledge about human exposure. Because of these, the actual prerequisites for extrapolation from high to low dose effects with the experimental data obtained and for extrapolation from species to species are still difficult to meet. Application of general mathematical models often leads to unacceptable variation in estimated incidences over several orders of magnitude.

Validation was discussed as another weak area of extrapolation. First, it should be pointed out that the significance and relevance of endpoints accessible by short-term tests for carcinogenicity are not well understood. Secondly, if one assumes the significance and relevance of an endpoint to exist, the validation process for this short-term test should comprise the assessment of its discriminative power, i.e., sensitivity in detecting true positive and negative results but avoiding false positive and negative ones. Such an assessment should be approached by testing not only compounds with known "carcinogenic" potential, but also – most particularly – those with unknown potential.

SESSION 3

Chemical Carcinogens: Primary Prevention

Chairman: D. Schmähl

Possibilities of Primary Prevention Against Chemical Carcinogens

R. Preussmann

The only promising strategy, in the foreseeable future, is to learn what are the causes of cancer and then to learn how to avoid them.

J. Cairns
Nature 300:398 (1982)

Principles of Primary Prevention

The fight against cancer is based on two strategies: cancer prevention and cancer treatment. Without doubt, there has been progress in the treatment of different types of cancer, but since estimated cures lie at around only 30%, cancer preventive measures evidently are of high priority. I therefore fully agree with John Cairns in stating that in the near future prevention will be the most successful strategy against cancer.

However, I want to emphasize that in spite of successful activities in the field of cancer prevention, new scientific results are not always (or often too slowly) put into practice and that in basic research not all working hypotheses are tested experimentally to the extent that they can be adapted and studied in humans. But in this respect perhaps the example of tobacco cancer exerts an inhibiting effect. The causes of tobacco cancer have been well known for a long time, but for a number of reasons no effective measures for risk prevention and elimination have been implemented by legislatures.

If primary prevention is defined as "elimination of hazardous factors before their becoming effective" (Roche Lexikon Medizin 1984), then it is obvious that the implementation of effective measures for cancer prevention depends directly upon the knowledge of the causes of cancer. From the three groups of carcinogenic risk factors, namely, chemical carcinogens, ionizing radiation, and oncogenic viruses, I will concentrate mainly on chemical carcinogens. This can be justified by the fact that research in the causes of cancer is still based on the concept that "environmental carcinogens" are responsible for the majority of human cancers. The carcinogenic effect of chemical carcinogens or mixtures of chemical carcinogens is determined by the following methods with decreasing evidential value:

1. Epidemiological investigations in man
2. Animal experiments
3. So-called short-term tests, especially for the determination of mutagenic effects

The importance of epidemiological data in man is evident. We assume that the results of proper animal experiments can usually be directly extrapolated to humans, with certain limitations. Short-term tests should and must be scrutinized very criti-

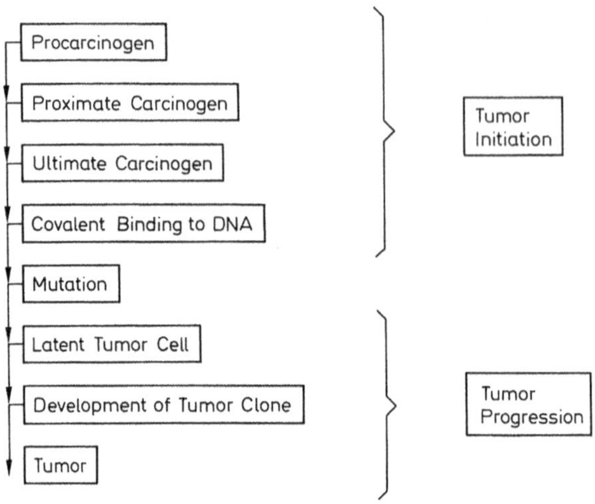

Fig. 1. Mechanism of carcinogenesis for genotoxic chemicals; proposed mechanism of activation

cally in respect to their relevance for carcinogenesis in man; the former euphoria ("carcinogens are mutagens"; Ames et al. 1973) has given way to the more sober estimation that only 65% of known carcinogens have been proven to be mutagens (Harper et al. 1983). For this reason, short-term tests can not yet replace animal experiments.

To outline the basic possibilities of primary prevention of cancer it is necessary to revert to the now widely accepted theory of chemical carcinogenesis by genotoxic carcinogens (Fig. 1).

After exposure of the organism to the carcinogenic agent, metabolic activation of so-called procarcinogenic compounds, which are not active per se but require in vivo activation by enzymatic processes, is a first step. It mainly consists of oxidative processes by microsomal mixed function oxidases (P-450 cytochrome) to give chemically reactive intermediates, the so-called proximal carcinogens. By further chemical and/or enzymatic processes, they are in turn transformed into the so-called ultimate carcinogen. This ultimate carcinogen is highly reactive (electrophilic) and interacts with nucleophiles in biological macromolecules to form stable adducts. If this happens in genetic material, such as DNA, the adduct formed is considered to be a point mutation which on cell replication will transfer false information leading to irreversible damage. This whole sequence is called *tumor initiation*. Latest experimental results show that by point mutations, proto-oncogenes or oncogenes can be activated in the genetic material. This might be the specific mechanism of tumor initiation (Zarbl et al. 1985).

Carcinogenesis by ionizing radiation falls easily into this scheme: radiation induces DNA alterations and thus mutations. Viral carcinogens change the genetic code of the cell by integration of viral DNA into the genetic material of mammalian cells.

The transformed cell known as a *latent tumor cell* then enters into a relatively slow growth phase (tumor progression) acting as a parent cell to give malignant clones and precancerous cells with specific biochemical and pathomorphological characteristics which ultimately result in macroscopically manifest tumors.

In the early phases of tumor progression, growth can be accelerated or inhibited by so-called promotors or inhibitors. For this reason it seems possible to put the end of primary prevention and the start of early detection (secondary prevention) into this phase and not at the end of initiation.

Prevention by Avoidance or Reduction of Exposure

Referring to the above statements, it is clear that a prevention of human exposure to cancer risk factors is the "most simple" way of primary prevention. It can clearly be stated that if complete avoidance of exposure is impossible, at least a reduction of the carcinogenic load has to be aimed for. Cancer epidemiology as well as experimental cancer research have shown clear-cut dose-response relationships, thus, lower exposure ultimately means lower risk.

For the implementation of preventive measures after detection of human risk factors, several principal methods are available. Without going into details, as these will be given in some of the following contributions, the following preventive measures are available:

1. Legal measures
2. Modified production techniques
3. Personal measures

Legal measures have been implemented to reduce the exposure to carcinogens in foodstuffs, air, and drinking water to a minimum. In addition to allowed maximum concentrations of food additives, carcinogenic food contaminants such as PAHs, aflatoxin, and nitrosamines have to be within a defined maximum permitted limit. Foodstuffs which exceed these limits have to be removed from the market.

In the field of air pollution, emission standards for certain carcinogens have recently been established by legal measures in the Federal Republic of Germany.

The system of legislative measures, necessary as it is, is not always used logically and consistently. Above all, the nonexistence of adequate legal measures against smoking is difficult to understand from a scientific point of view. In the food sector a maximum permitted level of polycyclic aromatic hydrocarbons in smoked meat products has been introduced in this country, but foodstuffs of plant origin are not covered although in the latter the concentration of these potent carcinogens may be higher by a factor of 500. Nitrate exposure from drinking water is legally restricted, however, the normally much higher load from certain types of vegetables is not regulated at all.

The area of production techniques is of great importance not only in the industrial sector, but also in agriculture (pesticides, fertilizers). Production has been halted (for example, β-naphthylamine and benzidine in chemical industries, PCB production), or production switched to the manufacture of alternative products with similar technological properties, but without the carcinogenic effects. Examples of the latter are the reduction of nitrosamine exposure in the rubber industry (Spiegelhalder and Preussmann 1983) and the exchange of polyvinyl chloride for polyethylene in food packaging.

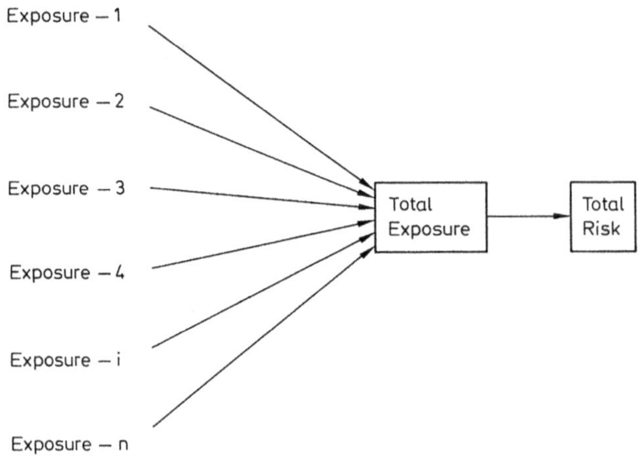

Fig. 2. Multicausal chemical carcinogenesis; scheme for risk estimation

If high-risk productions cannot be stopped, work has to be performed in closed systems with strict safety regulations for potentially exposed workers.

In the field of personal measures, nonsmoking would be one of the most logical and successful actions.

In regard to other environmental exposures, the individual might take countermeasures on the basis of reliable and not exaggerated information, e.g., by avoiding mould-contaminated foods. The strict observance of radiation protective measures against exposure to ionizing radiation has reduced the incidence of respective tumors in potentially exposed persons to almost zero.

The effectiveness of primary prevention measures by exposure prevention or reduction has been proven epidemiologically for monocausal cancer induction as, e.g., occupational cancers or quasimonocausal ones, like smoking. Much more difficult, if not impossible to obtain with the methods presently available in epidemiology, is similar evidence for a typical multicausal process like environmental carcinogenesis with many different but usually very low single exposures.

Here the concept is valid that the "total carcinogen load" of the individual is equal to the sum of single exposures and the total exposure corresponds to the total risk (Fig. 2). The elimination or reduction of single exposures will also reduce the total exposure and thus the risk of cancer. Such a process unfortunately is slow and can only be achieved one step at a time.

Intervention in the Phase of Carcinogen Activation

The metabolic changes necessary for activation of genotoxic carcinogens (Fig. 1) are not the only metabolic processes in vivo (Fig. 3). A series of *detoxifying* processes might in theory be used for prevention strategies. The following possibilities might be envisaged:

1. Interference at the stage of carcinogen metabolism
2. Scavenging of reactive ultimate carcinogens

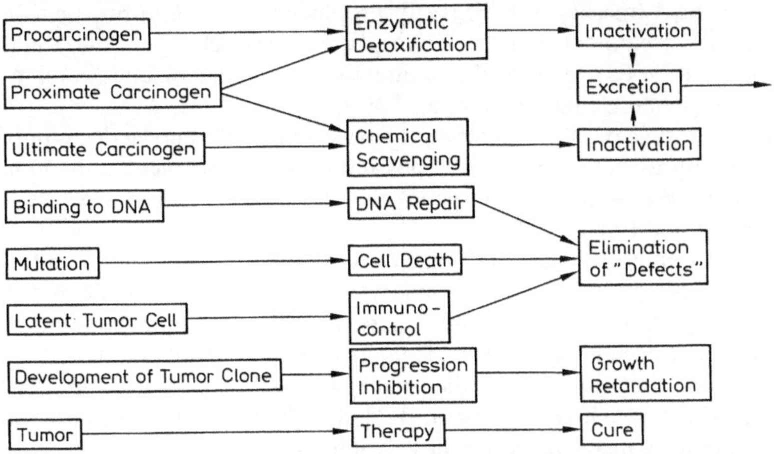

Fig. 3. Mechanism of carcinogenesis for genotoxic chemicals; possible inactivation processes

3. Interference at the stage of DNA repair processes
4. Influencing immune surveillance
5. Inhibition of tumor progression

Enzymatic processes can be stimulated as well as inhibited. To achieve an anticarcinogenic effect at the stage of the metabolism of chemical carcinogens in the mammalian organism, either activation processes should be inhibited and/or detoxifying processes should be stimulated. Mixed function oxidases can be strongly modified in their enzymatic activity and changed activities manifest themselves in different carcinogenic potencies. Examples for relevant enzyme modulators are some flavones, which inhibit the metabolism of polycyclic aromatic hydrocarbons, with the consequence of an inhibition of carcinogenicity of these substances in mouse experiments (Wattenberg 1978; Slaga and DiGiovanni 1984). This applies to naturally occurring as well as synthetic flavonoids. Another group of important enzyme inducers are polychlorinated hydrocarbons, e.g., PCBs, DDT, and dioxines. PCBs, for instance, inhibit skin carcinogenesis induced by dimethylbenzanthracene, liver carcinogenesis by aflatoxin, diethylnitrosamine, or acetaminofluorene (Slaga and DiGiovanni 1984).

A second approach is the blocking of interaction of reactive carcinogen metabolites with DNA as a presumptive critical target. In this respect, nucleophilic sulfur-containing compounds play an important part as anticarcinogens. The radioprotective potency of many of these substances has been known for some time (Bacq 1965); their effectiveness in radiation protection is well known. Cysteamine inhibits mammary carcinogenesis by DMBA in the rat (Marquardt et al. 1975), other effective inhibitors in animal experiments are disulfiram, dithiocarbamates, and benzylthiocyanate (Wattenberg 1978; Slaga and DiGiovanni 1984). The example of disulfiram and nitrosamine carcinogenesis shows clearly that combined application effectively inhibits liver carcinogenesis, but in combination experiments, esophageal tumors are observed, i.e., a change in organotropy took place (Schmähl et al. 1976).

2-Mercapto-sulfonic acid (mesna) is effective in prophylaxis of acute urotoxic side effects after cytostatic treatment with cyclophosphamide (Brock et al. 1982) and cisplatin (Kempf et al. 1985); mesna also inhibits experimental bladder carcinogenesis with cyclophosphamide (Schmähl et al. 1984).

Interference at the stage of DNA repair on the basis of present knowledge is only a theoretical possibility for intervention; the possibility of an influence on immune surveillance (Burnet 1964) is also highly speculative, because the concept per se is controversial (Kripke and Borsos 1974).

The inhibition of tumor growth in the stage of tumor progression is little understood from a mechanistic point of view. The issue, especially in regard to vitamin A and retinoids, is being intensely investigated in experiments and in epidemiology. A series of pilot studies, especially in smokers, is in progress in Finland and the USA.

Experimentally well investigated are the anticarcinogenic effects of some antioxidants like BHA (butylated hydroxyanisol), BHT (butylated hydroxytoluole), and selenium. Their inhibitory mechanisms are largely unknown.

In summary, there is the question of the *practical* value of anticarcinogenic substances in primary cancer prevention for humans. There are still too many unanswered questions to justify general applicability.

As yet, we do not know what amounts of carcinogenesis inhibitors are needed to show effects in man. By manipulating the carcinogen metabolism, an inhibition of carcinogenesis by a group of carcinogens might stimulate the activation of another class of carcinogens. Of great importance is the inherent toxicity of the inhibitors: vitamin A and its derivatives possess a substantial toxicity as limiting factors, BHA and selenium are suspected to be weak carcinogens. The persistent chlorinated hydrocarbons of DDT type are certainly not suitable for application in humans.

In my opinion "chemoprevention" on a large scale is not yet suitable or advisable for most types of multicausal carcinogenesis; a large number of scientific investigations are still required for a practical solution.

However, in respect to monocausal or quasimonocausal origins of cancer, there are some practical possibilities I would like to propose. Chemoprevention for inhibition of secondary tumors after cytostatic therapy in humans might be an appropriate model for a safe testing of this concept. These patients have a known exposure to carcinogenic alkylating agents, for instance, cyclophosphamide, cisplatin, or nitrosoureas; they have a high risk of secondary tumors with short latency periods and are under permanent medical control. A possible reduction of the risk of bladder cancer after cyclophosphamide therapy with mesna as inhibitor should be demonstrable epidemiologically in future.

For the high incidence of acute nonlymphocytic leukemia after nitrosourea therapy (Boice et al. 1983), an experimentally appropriate inhibitor should be chosen and its efficacy proven in a controlled clinical trial.

In summary, it can be stated that in primary prevention of cancer the possibilities are not yet exhausted. Experimentally tested methods of exposure prevention or reduction should be further improved. Chemoprevention is a new way, which, on the basis of experimental investigations, might have new potential for application in humans. Some of these possibilities are highly speculative, others are so far proven that in appropriate risk groups the efficacy of chemoprevention in humans can be tested in pilot projects.

References

Ames BN, Durston W, Yamasaki E, Lee F (1973) Carcinogens are mutagens. Proc Natl Acad Sci USA 70: 2281–2285

Bacq ZM (1965) Chemical protection against ionizing radiation. Thomas, Springfield, USA, p 79ff

Boice J, Greene MH, Killen JY, Ellenberg SS, Keehn RJ, McFadden E, Chen TT, Fraumeni JF (1983) Leukemia and preleukemia after adjuvant treatment of gastrointestinal cancer with semustine (Me-CCNU). N Engl J Med 309: 1079–1084

Brock N, Habs M, Pohl J, Schmähl D, Stekar J (1982) Mesna (Natrium-2-Mercaptoethansulfonat) Prophylaxe der akuten urotoxischen Nebenwirkungen sowie der kanzerogenen Spätfolgen von Cyclophosphamid und Ifosfamid. Therapiewoche 32: 4975–4996

Burnet FM (1964) Immunological factors in the process of carcinogenesis. Br Med Bull 20: 154–158

Harper BL, Pinkus SJ, Scott M, Ammenhauser M, Bang KM, Lowery M, Legator MS (1983) Correlation of NCI and IARC carcinogens with their mutagenicity in Salmonella. In: Castellani A (ed) The use of human cells for the evaluation of risk from phycial and chemical agents. Plenum, New York, pp 353–424

Kempf SR, Ivankovic S, Wiesler M, Schmähl D (1985) Effective prevention of nephrotoxicity of cisplatin (CDDP) by administration of sodium 2-mercaptoethanesulfonate (Mesna) in rats. Br J Cancer 52: 937–939

Kripke ML, Borsos T (1974) Immune surveillance revisited. JNCI 52: 1393–1395

Marquardt H, Sapozink MD, Zedek M (1975) Inhibition by systeamine-HCl of oncogenesis induced by 7,12-dimethyl-benz(a)anthracene. JNCI 55: 653–657

Roche Lexikon Medizin (1984) Urban and Schwarzenberg, München, p 1290

Schmähl D, Habs M, Tacchi AM (1984) Prophylaxe der Tumorentstehung in der Harnblase durch Natrium-2-Mercaptoethansulfonat (Mesna). Urologe [Ausg A] 23: 291–296

Schmähl D, Krüger FW, Habs M, Diehl B (1976) Influence of disulfiram on the organotropy of the carcinogenic effect of dimethylnitrosamine and diethylnitrosamine in rats. Z Krebsforsch 85: 271–272

Slaga TJ, DiGiovanni J (1984) Inhibition of chemical carcinogenesis. In: Searle CE (ed) Chemical carcinogens. American Chemical Society, Washington, DC, pp 1279–1321

Spiegelhalder B, Preussmann R (1983) Occupational nitrosamine exposure. 1. Rubber and tyre industry. Carcinogenesis 4: 1147–1152

Wattenberg LW (1978) Inhibitors of chemical carcinogenesis. Adv Cancer Res 26: 197–226

Zarbl H, Sukumar S, Arthur AV, Martin-Zanca D, Barbacid M (1985) Direct mutagenesis of HA-ras-oncogens by N-nitroso-N-methylurea during initiation of mammary carcinogenesis in rats. Nature 315: 382–385

Primary Prevention Against Occupational Carcinogens

P. J. LANDRIGAN and I. J. SELIKOFF

Introduction

Cancer kills approximately 430000 people in the United States of America each year. The American Cancer Society estimates that some form of cancer will develop in one-fourth of all Americans (American Cancer Society 1985). It is the second leading cause of death and the second leading cause of lost years of potential life in the United States of America (Centers for Disease Control 1983).

Considerable progress toward cancer control has stemmed from the recognition that chemical agents can cause cancer. Percivall Pott (1775) reported for the first time an association between cancer and an environmental agent. Pott noted that the "climbing boys" of London, teenage lads and young men employed as chimney sweeps, experienced a devastating incidence of cancer of the scrotum. He attributed the development of those tumors to exposure to soot. Subsequently, Rehn (1895) noted a high frequency of cancer of the urinary bladder among workers in the aniline dye industry. He attributed the etiology of those tumors to occupational exposure to aromatic amines. More recently, etiologic associations have been recognized between benzene and leukemia (Delore and Borgomano 1928); asbestos and lung cancer (Lynch and Smith 1935); arsenic and cancer of the skin, lung, and liver (Hill and Faning 1948); bis-chloromethyl ether and lung cancer (Figueroa et al. 1973); and vinyl chloride monomer and angiosarcoma of the liver (Creech and Johnson 1974). Most importantly in terms of the number of persons affected, cigarette smoking has been found to cause cancer of the lungs, bladder, larynx, and esophagus (Doll and Hill 1956) (Table 1).

Toxicologic studies stimulated by those clinical and epidemiologic observations have led to fundamental advances in the understanding of the biology of cancer. Benzo[a]pyrene, a polynuclear aromatic hydrocarbon compound found in soot, has been found to induce skin cancer in experimental animals (Kenneway 1924); that provides a molecular basis for Pott's observations of the link between soot and scrotal cancer. Likewise, β-naphthylamine, a chemical intermediary in aniline dye manufacturing, has been shown to cause cancer of the bladder in experimental animals (Hueper et al. 1938), thus providing an experimental explanation for the observations of Rehn (1895). Additionally, each of these compounds has been found capable of reacting with DNA in exposed cells so as to alter the structure of the double helix and thus cause errors in DNA replication (Weinstein 1981). Somatic mutations can result, and one consequence of certain somatic mutations is malignant transformation. The understanding of such mechanisms constitutes a major step towards development of a biochemical basis for the control of cancer.

Table 1. Selected occupational cancers (adapted from Rutstein et al. 1983)

ICD-9[a]	Condition	Industry/occupation	Agent
155	Hemangiosarcoma of the liver	Vinyl chloride polymerization Industry Vintners	Vinyl chloride monomer Arsenical pesticides
160.0	Malignant neoplasm of nasal cavities	Woodworkers, cabinet/ furniture makers Boot and shoe producers Radium chemists, processors, dial painters, nickel smelting and refining	Hardwood dusts Unknown Radium Nickel
161	Malignant neoplasm of larynx	Asbestos industries and utilizers	Asbestos
158	Mesothelioma (peritoneum; pleural)	Asbestos industries and utilizers	Asbestos
170	Malignant neoplasm of bone	Radium chemists, processors, dial painters	Radium
187.7	Malignant neoplasm of scrotum	Automatic lathe operators, metalworkers Coke oven workers, petroleum refiners, tar distillers	Mineral/cutting oils Soots and tars, tar distillates
188	Malignant neoplasm of bladder	Rubber and dye workers	Benzidine, α- and β-naphthylamine, auramine, magenta, 4-aminobiphenyl, 4-nitrophenyl
189	Malignant neoplasm of kidney and unspecified urinary organs	Coke oven workers	Coke oven emissions
204	Lymphoid leukemia, acute	Rubber industry, radiologists	Unknown, ionizing radiation
205	Myeloid leukemia, acute	Occupations with exposure to benzene, radiologists	Benzene
207.0	Erythroleukemia	Occupations with exposure to benzene	Benzene

[a] Modified International Classification of Diseases (ICD) rubric

The recognition of environmental carcinogenesis has had a profound influence on the study of cancer epidemiology. No longer must cancer be regarded as an inescapable consequence of aging. Instead, it is now realized that chemical carcinogenesis is not exceptional, and that well over half of human cancers – perhaps as many as 80%–90% worldwide – are caused by environmental exposure to carcinogens (Higginson and Muir 1979). Such "environmental factors" are considered to include not only exposure to industrial chemicals and pollutants, but also such other influences as diet, alcohol, tobacco, drugs, radiation, and sexual behavior. The most stimulating implication of the environmental cancer hypothesis is the notion it entails that a very high proportion of all human cancer ought to be preventable by the conceptually simple practice of reducing exposure to environmental carcinogens.

Occupational Etiology of Cancer

The extent to which occupational factors contribute to the etiology of human cancer remains uncertain. Several intrinsic characteristics contribute to the difficulty of making estimates of the proportion of cancer which is attributable to occupational exposure. These factors include the following:

- The long latency which typically elapses between exposure to carcinogen and development of cancer
- Disentangling exposures to multiple carcinogens
- The confounding influence of behavioral factors, such as cigarette smoking. This issue is complicated further by the fact that various behavioral factors may interact with chemical and physical agents in the working environment to increase the risk of cancer substantially (Table 1)

In addition, problems in the diagnosis and reporting of cancer and in the documentation of the nature and extent of past occupational exposures may obscure important epidemiologic associations. These issues can make the delineation of dose-response relationships between occupational exposure and cancer an exceptionally difficult task (Landrigan et al. 1985).

Despite these difficulties, several attempts have been made to estimate the proportion of cancers which are related to occupational exposure. These estimates span a broad range from less than 4% (Doll and Peto 1981; Higginson and Muir 1976) to more than 20% US Department of Health, Education, and Welfare 1978). Differences in definitions of populations at risk and differences in the assessment of carcinogenic exposures are among the factors which account for much of this variation (Davis et al. 1982; Selikoff 1981).

This variation notwithstanding, virtually all authors in the field of occupational carcinogenesis agree on the following two points:

Table 2. Age-standardized lung cancer death rates[a] for cigarette smoking and/or occupational exposure to asbestos dust compared with no smoking and no exposure (Hammond et al. 1979)

Group	Exposure to asbestos?	History of cigarette smoking	Death rate	Mortality difference	Mortality ratio
Control	No	No	11.3	0.0	1.00
Asbestos workers	Yes	No	58.4	+47.1	5.17
Control	No	Yes	122.6	+111.3	10.85
Asbestos workers	Yes	Yes	601.6	+590.3	53.24

[a] Rate per 100000 man-years standardized for age on the distribution of the man-years of all the asbestos workers. Number of lung cancer deaths based on death certificate information

- The incidence of occupational cancer falls especially heavily on certain population subgroups. For example, among long-term benzene workers, the relative risk of death from leukemia is over 30 times background (Rinsky et al. 1981). Among asbestos workers who also smoke, the relative risk of lung cancer is greater than 50 times background (Hammond et al. 1979) (Table 2). Finally, among certain populations of workers exposed to benzidine and β-naphthylamine, over 80% have died of cancer of the bladder (Parkes 1978)
- Occupational cancer is highly preventable

Primary Prevention of Occupational Cancer

Primary prevention is defined in public health terminology as etiologic prevention, i.e., as prevention which is directed against the source of disease. A classic example from the field of infectious disease epidemiology is vaccination against poliomyelitis. Primary prevention contrasts with later (secondary and tertiary) forms of prevention which involve, respectively, the early detection of disease and the treatment of disease to prevent death. Examples of secondary prevention include the removal of a toxin which has already been released into the environment, medical screening of exposed persons to detect early disease, or behavioral modification. A classic example of tertiary prevention from infectious disease epidemiology is the use of the iron lung to prevent death in persons already infected with the poliomyelitis virus. Primary prevention is inherently more efficient and effective than secondary or tertiary prevention.

Several avenues exist for the primary prevention of occupational cancer.

Premarket Toxicologic Screening. Evaluation of the toxicology of new chemical compounds prior to their commercial release constitutes a most effective means for preventing cancer and other forms of human toxicity. Such assessment can include review of structure-activity relations, the application of short-term tests, or animal bioassays. It is important that such tests be universally and systematically applied and that resulting data be publicly available.

A major study conducted in the United States of America by the National Academy of Sciences (1984) demonstrates unfortunately that the majority of chemicals cur-

Table 3. Test data on the carcinogenicity of chemicals in the United States of America (US National Academy of Sciences 1984)

Category	Number	Availability of data permitting assessment of possible carcinogenic risk		
		% good data	% partial data	% no data
Pesticides	3350	10	33	38
Drugs	1815	18	33	25
Food additives	8627	5	18	46
Cosmetics	3410	2	12	56
Commercial chemicals	49000	0	10	78

rently in commerce have not received adequate premarket screening for carcinogenesis. Indeed, despite the passage in 1976 of the Toxic Substances Control Act, there are many thousands of chemicals currently on the market which have received no premarket screening (Table 3). Additionally, even for new compounds, testing requirements for carcinogenesis have not yet been standardized and responsibility for deciding whether to assess carcinogenicity, as well as responsibility for deciding which tests to perform, is left principally with the chemical manufacturers. In the United States of America, governmental review of the carcinogenic potential consists typically only of examination of their structural chemical formulae.

Industrial Hygiene. A second approach to the primary prevention of occupational cancer consists of the application of techniques derived from industrial hygiene.

Most efficient of these techniques is the *substitution* of a new, less hazardous material for a material of known carcinogenicity. It is, however, most important to ensure that the new material is indeed less hazardous than that which it replaces.

Another technique derived from industrial hygiene is that of *process enclosure.* This approach has been employed widely in the nuclear industry.

A third such approach consists of *ventilation.* The most effective ventilation is that which is applied at the source of generation of an airborne fume or particulate. General ventilation of a workroom area is a less effective technique.

A fourth approach consists of equipping workers with *personal protective equipment.* Such equipment can be indispensable in certain circumstances, as with short-term repairs, breakdowns, or during unusual operations. However, the extended use of personal protective equipment does not constitute an adequate approach to the control of occupational carcinogenic hazards.

Legal and Administrative Approaches. In the primary prevention of occupational cancer legal initiatives have been extremely effective. Among these are the banning of a chemical, for example, banning Kepone from commerce in the United States of America; the setting of an extremely stringent exposure standard which makes use of the chemical impractical, such as that regulating occupational exposure to chrysotile asbestos in Great Britain; the structural linking of worker compensation fees to the actual costs of disease so that employers can no longer avoid paying those costs; tort legislation in which workers are empowered to sue the manufacturers of hazardous material for injuries suffered; and finally criminal sanctions, under which employers may be fined or imprisoned in situations in which they have knowingly and recklessly exposed workers to occupational carcinogens or other toxins. Virtually all developed nations have adopted mixes of these legal and administrative strategies, although the combinations vary considerably from one nation to another in keeping with wide variations in legal tradition (Tchertkoff and Selikoff 1947).

Epidemiologic Surveillance. Another approach to the primary prevention of occupational cancer involves epidemiologic surveillance. Although, by definition, epidemiologic studies require that disease or death must have already occurred in a population, nevertheless, the detection by epidemiologic means of occupationally induced cancer provides a powerful basis for the prevention of future cases. A particular advantage of this approach is that it has the potential to detect carcinogenicity resulting from multiple factor interactions. For example, it is unlikely that the interaction between cigarette smoke and asbestos fibers in the etiology of lung cancer would have been detected except through epidemioligc study (Table 2).

Application of "Biological Markers." In the future biological markers will likely provide a new mechanism for the primary prevention of cancer (Weinstein 1981). "Markers" constitute biological, cytogenetic, physiologic, or other natural changes which result from exposure to a carcinogen and appear to presage in some fashion the development of cancer. The application of markers to the early detection of cancer will produce several gains, as follows: (a) the earlier detection than heretofore of environmentally induced cancers; (b) the detection of a larger percentage of affected persons than currently is possible; (c) the detection of premalignant change at low levels of exposure; and (d) the possibility of early treatment or early interruption of exposure before irreversible malignant cellular transformation has occurred. Additionally, the use of newly developed "markers" of chemical exposure will permit more precise assessment of past exposures, clearer delineation of exposure-effect relations, and better delineation of disease mechanisms, particularly at low dose levels. The application of such techniques in epidemiologic studies of populations exposed to occupational carcinogens is expected to lead to substantial increases in the understanding of the etiology of occupational cancer.

Conclusions

Cancer caused by occupational agents is a problem of human origin and should, therefore, be highly preventable. Primary prevention of occupational cancer may be achieved by means of a combination of techniques, including premarket toxicologic testing of new chemical compounds, application of industrial hygiene techniques, legal and regulatory approaches, epidemiologic surveillance, and the augmentation of epidemiologic surveillance through application of "biological markers."

Age-adjusted mortality rates for cancer in the United States of America have shown a slow but steady increase over the past several decades, and there is no evidence of a recent reversal (Bailar and Smith 1986). The extent to which occupationally induced cancer contributes to this overall trend is uncertain. However, the increased volume and diversity of synthetic chemicals manufactured since World War II raises serious concern about the cumulative population risks of exposure to these substances (Davis and Magee 1979). Reversal of present trends in cancer incidence will require ever more vigorous application of the techniques of primary prevention. The most efficient of these is premarket toxicologic screening of new chemical compounds, an approach which heretofore has been insufficiently applied (National Research Council 1984).

References

American Cancer Society (1985) Cancer statistics, 1985. CA 35:19–56
Bailar JC, Smith EM (1986) Progress against cancer? N Engl J Med 314:1226–1232

Centers for Disease Control (1983) Years of potential life lost, deaths, and death rates by cause of death, and estimated number of physician contacts, by principal diagnosis, US. MMWR 32:411
Creech JL Jr, Johnson MN (1974) Angioscarcoma of the liver in the manufacture of polyvinyl chloride. J Occup Med 16:150–151
Davis DL, Magee BH (1979) Cancer and industrial chemical production. Science 206:1356–1358
Davis DL, Bridbord K, Schneiderman M (1982) Cancer prevention: assessing causes, exposures, and recent trends in mortality for U.S. males, 1968–1978. Teratog Carcinog Mutag 2:105–135
Delore P, Borgomano C (1928) Acute leukemia following benzene poisoning. On the toxic origin of certain acute leukemias and their relation to serious anemias. J Med Lyon 9:227–233
Doll R, Hill AB (1956) Lung cancer and other causes of death in relation to smoking – a second report on the mortality of British doctors. Br Med J 2:1071–1077
Doll R, Peto R (1981) The causes of cancer: quantitative estimates of avoidable risks of cancer in the United States today. JNCI 66:1191–1265
Figueroa WG, Raszowski R, Weiss W (1973) Lung cancer in chloromethyl methyl ether workers. N Engl J Med 228:1096–1097
Hammond EC, Selikoff IJ, Churg J (1968) Asbestos exposure, smoking and neoplasia. JAMA 204(2):106–112
Hammond EC, Selikoff IJ, Seidman H (1979) Asbestos exposure, cigarette smoking and death rates. Ann NY Acad Sci 330:473–490
Higginson J, Muir CS (1976) The role of epidemiology in elucidating the importance of environmental factors in human cancer. Cancer Detect Prev 1:79–105
Higginson J, Muir CS (1979) Environmental carcinogenesis: misconceptions and limitations to cancer control. JNCI 63:1291–1298
Hill AB, Faning EL (1948) Studies in the incidence of cancer in a factory handling inorganic compounds of arsenic: I. Mortality experience in the factory. Br J Ind Med 5:1–6
Hueper WC, Wiley FH, Wolfe HD (1938) Experimental production of bladder tumors in dogs by administration of beta-naphtylamine. J Ind Hyg 20:46–84
Kenneway EL (1924) On the cancer-producing factor in tar. Br Med J 1:564–567
Landrigan PJ, Melius JM, Rinsky RA, Thum MJ (1985) Approaches to the estimation of exposure in occupational epidemiology. Banbury Rep Risk quantitation and regulatory policy 19:65–78
Lynch KM, Smith WA (1935) Pulmonary asbestosis: III. Carcinoma of lung increases asbesto-silicosis. Am J Cancer 24:56
National Academy of Sciences (1984) Toxicity testing: strategies to determine needs and priorities. National Academy Press, Washington, D.C.
Parkes HG (1978) Identification of carcinogenic hazards from aromatic amine exposure and measures of control. In: Nieburg HE (ed) Prevention and detection of cancer, part I. Dekker, New York
Pott P (1775) Chirurgical observations relative to the cataract, the polypus of the nose, the cancer of the scrotum, the different kinds of ruptures, and the mortification of the toes and feet. Hewes, Clarke and Collins, London
Rehn L (1895) Blasengeschwuelste bei Fuchsinarbeitern. Arch Klin Chur 50:588–600
Rinsky RA, Young RJ, Smith HE (1981) Leukemia in benzene workers. Am J Ind Med 2:217–245
Rutstein DD, Mullan RJ, Frazier TM, Halperin WE, Melius JM, Sestito AP (1983) Sentinel health events (occupational): a basis for physician recognition in public health surveillance. Am J Public Health 73:1054–1062
Selikoff IJ (1981) Constraints in estimating occupational contributions to current cancer mortality in the United States. In: Moran LA (ed) Quantification of occupational cancer (Banbury Rep 9). Cold Spring Harbor, New York, pp 3–17
Tchertkoff IG, Selikoff IJ (1947) The role of traumatism in the induction of initial pneumothorax: further studies. Q Bull Sea View Hosp 9:1–20
US Dept Health Education and Welfare (1978) Estimates of the fraction of cancer in the United States related to occupational factors. National Cancer Institute, National Institute of Environmental Health Sciences, National Institute for Occupational Safety and Health, Bethesda
Weinstein IB (1981) The scientific basis for carcinogen detection and primary cancer prevention. Cancer 47:1133–1141

Chemical Carcinogens in Tobacco*

D. Hoffmann, E. L. Wynder, S. S. Hecht, K. D. Brunnemann, E. J. LaVoie, and N. J. Haley

Introduction

The association of tobacco usage and cancer has been known for more than five decades. Clinical observations by F. H. Mueller in Cologne in 1939 and by Schairer and Schoeniger in Jena in 1943 were among the first reports to indicate an increased risk for lung cancer among smokers. However, it was not until 1950 that the evidence from case-control studies in the UK and the USA directed attention towards the association of cigarette smoking with lung cancer (Doll and Hill 1950; Levin et al. 1950; Wynder and Graham 1950). In the following 35 years, more than 100 epidemiological reports from at least 15 countries have formed the basis for the conclusions of the US Surgeon General (1982), the Royal College of Physicians (1983), and the International Agency for Research on Cancer (IARC 1986) that cigarette smoking is causally associated with cancer of the lung, larynx, oral cavity, and esophagus, and correlated with cancer of the pancreas, kidney, and urinary bladder, and, possibly also with cancer of the cervix. Cigar and pipe smoking are also causally associated with cancer of the lung, larynx, oral cavity, and esophagus, although the association of these tobacco habits with cancer of the lung and of the larynx is less strong than that of cigarette smoking. Passive smoking gives rise to some risk of cancer (IARC 1986). It has also been concluded that oral use of snuff is carcinogenic to humans (IARC 1985; US Surgeon General 1986).

Bioassays

Most of the epidemiological observations on tobacco exposure and cancer have been convincingly supported by laboratory studies (Wynder and Hoffmann 1967; Mohr and Reznik 1978). Whole cigarette smoke induces benign and malignant tumors of the larynx in Syrian golden hamsters (Dontenwill et al. 1973; Bernfeld et al. 1974) and tumors of the lung in rats and mice (Mohr and Reznik 1978; Dalbey et al. 1980), however, the gas phase of cigarette smoke produces only adenoma and adenocarcinoma of the lung in the mouse (Leuchtenberger and Leuchtenberger 1970). The particulate matter of the smoke of cigarettes, cigars, and pipes induces benign and malignant tumors in the skin of mice and rabbits, the connective tissue of rats, the lung of rats, and the cervix of mice (Wynder and Hoffmann 1967; Mohr and Reznik 1978).

* Our tobacco research program is supported by U.S. National Cancer Institute grant P01-CA-29580

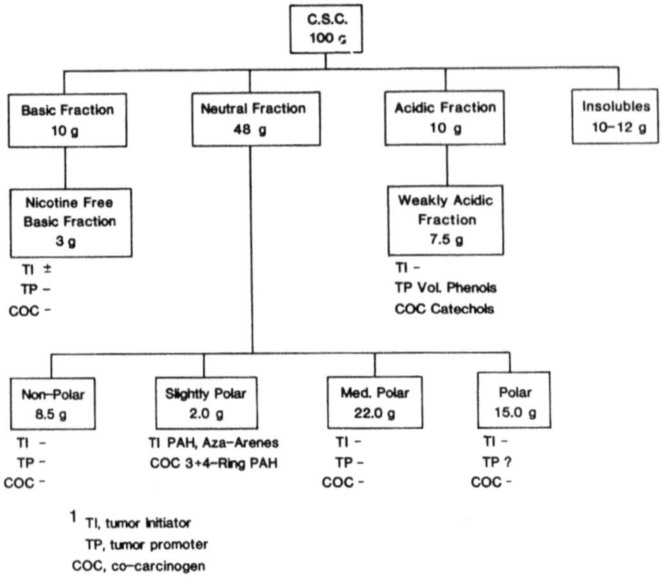

Fig. 1. Fractionation of cigarette smoke condensate

The unique assets of the laboratory studies lie in their capabilities to identify tumorigenic and carcinogenic compounds in a complex environmental matrix and to determine their biological mode of action. The understanding of the nature and biochemical functions of the tumorigenic agents is requisite towards an approach for reducing or eliminating the carcinogenicity of an environmental agent.

In the case of the particulate matter of tobacco smoke, in-depth fractionation studies have led to the identification of tumor initiators, tumor promoters, and cocarcinogens (Hoffmann and Wynder 1971; Bock et al. 1971; Hecht et al. 1975; Van Duuren and Goldschmidt 1976; Hecht et al. 1981). Figure 1 summarizes our present knowledge about the nature of the tumorigenic agents in tobacco smoke condensate according to bioassays on the skin of mice and rabbits. The major tumor initiators in smoke particulates are certain types of polynuclear aromatic hydrocarbons (PAH) and aza-arenes which reside in the slightly polaric neutral subfractions. Tumor promoters identified thus far include semivolatile phenols in the weakly acidic fractions, and still unidentified compounds in the polaric neutral subfraction. The major known cocarcinogens in the condensate are catechols, which are the most abundant phenolic compounds in the smoke and, in the neutral slightly polaric fraction, certain 3- and 4-ring PAH.

Reduction in Tumorigenicity

Inhalation studies carried out with Syrian golden hamsters exposed to whole cigarette smoke, and bioassays of smoke condensate on mouse skin have clearly demonstrated that a significant reduction of particulate matter and of PAH leads to a con-

Table 1. Relative effectiveness of techniques used commercially in the United States for reducing the biological activity of cigarette smoke

Methods	Smoke constituents[a]			Biological activity[b]	
	Tar	Nicotine	BaP	Carcinogenicity	Tumor promotion
Agriculture					
Tobacco type (bright-burley)	+	+	+	+	+
New cultivars	+	+	+		?
Nitrate fertilization	+	+	+	+	?
Processing					
Cut	±	±	±	±?	?
Use of stems	+	+	+	++	++
RTS-nonpaper process[c]	+	+	+	++	±
RTS-paper process	++	+	+	++	±
Expanded tobacco	+	++	+	+	+
Expanded stems	+	++	+	++	?
Production					
Paper porosity	+	+	+	±	?
Cellulose acetate filters[d]	+	+	+	±	±
Charcoal filters[d]	+	+	+	±	±
Perforated filters	++	++	++	±	?

[a] Reductions: ++, >50%; +, significant; ±, insignificant; ±?, questionable; ?, unknown
[b] Comparison of gram to gram tar in mouse skin tests and/or hamster smoke inhalations
[c] Some RTS produce high levels of CO_2
[d] Reductions of tar, nicotine, and BaP (and other nonvolatiles), and volatile N-nitrosamines are in general, somewhat greater with cellulose acetate filters than with charcoal filters
BaP, benzo(a)pyrene; RTS, reconstituted tobacco sheets

comitant reduction of the tumorigenic potential of cigarette smoke (Wynder and Hoffmann 1961; Hoffmann and Wynder 1972; Dontenwill 1974; Dontenwill et al. 1977; Hoffmann et al. 1980). Methods that lead to the reduction of benzo(a)pyrene (BaP) and other PAH include selection of tobacco type, such as Burley varieties, special processing of the cigarette tobacco blend, such as adding reconstituted tobacco, expanded tobacco and stems, and the utilization of special cigarette wrappers and filter tips (Table 1). Some reduction of the tumor-promoting activity can be achieved by adding a high percentage of tobacco stems to the cigarette filler; however, changes in tobacco processing are generally more effective in reducing complete carcinogenicity than in diminishing tumor-promoting activity when these biological activities are measured on mouse skin. Manufacture of many of the present-day cigarettes in Western Europa and North America is now incorporating a number of such changes in processing aimed at reduction of smoke yields as well as modification of smoke composition.

Although these approaches towards the reduction of the carcinogenic potential of cigarette smoke were deemed of some practical value, they have not been widely accepted in the scientific community for a number of reasons. The reduction of tumorigenicity under laboratory conditions does not fully reflect the human setting. This is apparent from several studies which have shown that smokers of low-yield cigarettes tend to compensate for the lower nicotine and tar delivery by smoking more intensely (Herning et al. 1981; Haley et al. 1985). Nevertheless, a number of case-control studies have indicated that compared to a smoker of nonfilter cigarettes, the long-term smoker of low-yield cigarettes has a reduced risk for lung cancer. A working group of the International Agency for Research on Cancer (IARC 1986) concluded recently that "No substantial cause (or cofactor) has so far been identified that offers a plausible explanation for the observed magnitude of the reduction of risk for lung cancer, other than changes in cigarette design which include reduction in tar content." Then again, it needs to be stated that the substantial decreases in lung cancer mortality which have recently been observed in middle-aged groups in the United Kingdom and Finland, have not been seen in other countries. Perhaps this is due to the fact that the smoking habits, which were initiated when these European cohorts were young adults, became established long before the major reductions in smoke yields of cigarettes occurred (IARC 1986).

A concern of public health scientists relates to the fact that the smoker of low-yield cigarettes may be misled in regard to risk reduction, since the health benefits from cessation of smoking really vastly exceed those to be expected from changes in the design of the cigarette. Another concern is that the effect of changes in cigarette design on the smoker's risk of cancer at sites other than the lung and larynx have thus far not been evaluated. It must also be cited that data in respect to myocardial infarction and the low-yield cigarette are conflicting (US Surgeon General 1983). Finally, there is an uncertainty as to how flavor-enhancing additives in low-yield cigarettes may affect the biological activity of the smoke (LaVoie et al. 1985).

Organ-Specific Carcinogens

As discussed earlier, cigarette smoking is also correlated with cancer of the esophagus, pancreas, kidney, and urinary bladder, and possibly with cancer of the cervix (IARC 1986). This observation suggests the presence of organ-specific carcinogens in cigarette smoke (Table 2). Aromatic amines such as 2-naphthylamine and 4-aminobiophenyl, are known human bladder carcinogens and their presence in cigarette smoke has been considered as a contributing factor to the increased risk of cigarette smokers for bladder cancer (Doll 1971).

Other organ-specific carcinogens identified thus far are benzene, vinyl chloride, volatile nitrosamines, traces of metals, and polonium-210 (IARC 1986; Hoffmann and Wynder 1986). In respect to the organ-specific carcinogens we have directed much of our own research towards elucidating how nicotine, the major habituating agent in tobacco, contributes to the carcinogenic potential of tobacco products. Figure 2 presents nicotine and other alkaloids as precursors of the tobacco-specific N-nitrosamines (TSNA; Hoffmann and Hecht 1985). The TSNA are formed during the processing of tobacco (curing, fermentation, aging) and during smoking. Nicotine gives rise to *N'*-nitrosonornicotine (NNN), and to 4-(methylnitrosamino)-1-(3-pyridyl)-1-butanone (NNK). The nitrosation of the group of secondary tobacco alkaloids leads in the case of nornicotine to NNN, anatabine to *N'*-nitrosoanatabine (NAT), and in the

Table 2. Organ-specific carcinogens in the smoke of nonfilter cigarettes

Compound	Amount/cigarette	Evidence for carcinogenicity[a]	
		Humans	Animals
A. *Vapor phase*			
Benzene	12–48 μg	S	S
Hydrazine	32 ng	I	S
Formaldehyde[b]	70–100 μg		S
Vinyl chloride	1–16 ng	S	S
Acrylonitrile	3.2–15 μg	L	S
2-Nitropropane	0.73–1.21 μg		S
Nitrosodimethylamine	10–40 ng		S
Nitrosodiethylamine	0.0–10 ng		S
Nitrosopyrrolidine	6–30 ng		S
B. *Particulate phase*			
2-Toluidine	30–200 ng	I	S
4-Aminobiphenyl	2–5 ng	S	S
1-Naphthylamine	3–4 ng	I	I
2-Naphthylamine	1–22 ng	S	S
Arsenic	1–25 μg	S	I
Nickel	0.0–600 ng	L	S
Cadmium	9–70 ng	L	S
Polonium-210	0.04–0.1 pCi	Carc.[c]	Carc.[c]

[a] Degree of evidence for carcinogenicity according to IARC (1986)
[b] May be contact carcinogen
[c] Not reviewed by IARC, but known carcinogen in humans and animals
S, sufficient; L, limited evidence; I, inadequate

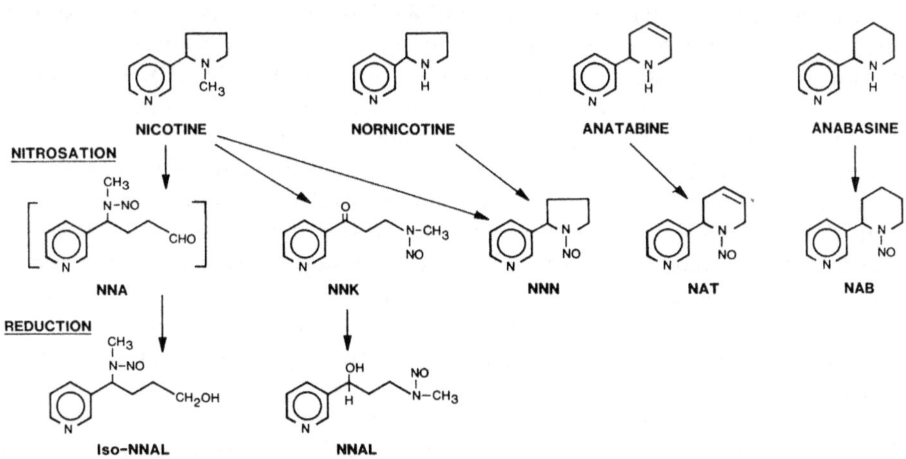

Fig. 2. Formation of tobacco-specific N-nitrosamines

Table 3. Carcinogenicity of tobacco-specific nitrosamines (TSNA; from Hoffmann and Hecht 1985)

Nitros-amine	Species and strains	Route of appli-cation	Principal target organs	Dose
NNK	A/J mouse	i.p.	Lung	0.12 mmol/mouse
	F344 rat	s.c.	Nasal cavity, liver, lung	0.1–2.8 mmol/rat
	Syrian golden hamster	s.c.	Trachea, lung, nasal cavity	0.005–0.9 mmol/hamster
NNN	A/J mouse	i.p.	Lung	0.12 mmol/mouse
	F344 rat	s.c.	Nasal cavity, esophagus	0.2–3.4 mmol/rat
	F344 rat	p.o.	Nasal cavity, esophagus	1.0–3.6 mmol/rat
	Sprague-Dawley rat	p.o.	Nasal cavity	8.8 mmol/rat
	Syrian golden hamster	s.c.	Trachea, nasal cavity	0.9–2.1 mmol/hamster
NAT	F344 rat	s.c.	None	0.2–2.8 mmol/rat
NAB	F344 rat	p.o.	Esophagus	3–12 mmol/rat
	Syrian golden hamster	s.c.	None	2 mmol/hamster
NNA	A/J mouse	i.p.	None	0.12 mmol/mouse
NNAL	A/J mouse	i.p.	Lung	0.12 mmol/mouse
Iso-NNAL	F344 rat	s.c.	? Under test	

Abbreviations for TSNA: NNK, 4-(methylnitrosamino)-1-(3-pyridyl)-1-butanone; NNN, *N'*-nitrosornonicotine; NAT, *N'*-nitrosoanatabine; NAB, *N'*-nitrosoanabasine; NNA, 4-(methylnitrosamino)-4-(3-pyridyl)butanal; NNAL, 4-(methylnitrosamino)-1-(3-pyridyl)-1-butanol; Iso-NNAL, 4-(methylnitrosamino)-4-(3-pyridyl)butanol

case of anabasine to *N'*-nitrosoanabasine (NAB). The oxidative N-nitrosation of nicotine would be expected to give rise not only to NNN and NNK, but also to 4-(methylnitrosamino)-4-(3-pyridyl)butanal (NNA). We have not detected this nitrosamino aldehyde in tobacco products, but have found its reduction product, the primary alcohol 4-(methylnitrosamino)-4-(3-pyridyl)-1-butanol (Iso-NNAL). Reduction of NNK leads to the corresponding secondary alcohol 4-(methylnitrosamino)-1-(3-pyridyl)-1-butanol (NNAL; Fig. 2; Brunnemann et al. 1987).

Of the six identified tobacco-specific nitrosamines we found NNN and NNK to be powerful carcinogens in mice, rats, and hamsters (Hoffmann and Hecht 1985). A single dose of 1 mg NNK induces a significant incidence of tumors in the respiratory tract of hamsters and, on a molar basis, NNK is a more powerful carcinogen in rats than N-nitrosodimethylamine (Hecht et al. 1986). NAB and NNAL are moderately active carcinogens; Iso-NNAL, which was only recently identified, is now being tested for tumorigenicity. NAT was inactive in rats at dose levels up to 9 mmol/kg (Table 3).

Perhaps the most important observation is that of the high concentrations of the TSNA (Table 4). In the case of snuff tobacco, which is a known human carcinogen when used orally, the nitrosamines exceed by at least two orders of magnitude the

Table 4. Tobacco-specific nitrosamines in commercial US tobacco products

Tobacco product	NNN	NNK	NAT + NAB
A. *Smokeless tobacco*			
Chewing tobacco (ppb)	3500–8200	100–3000	500–7000
Snuff (ppb)	800–89000	200–8300	200–4000
B. *Mainstream smoke*			
Cigarettes-NF (ng/cigarette)	120–950	80–770	140–990
Cigarettes-F (ng/cigarette)	50–310	30–150	60–370
Little cigar-F (ng/cigar)	5500	4200	1700
Cigar (ng/cigar)	3200	1900	1900
C. *Sidestream smoke*			
Cigarettes-NF (ng/cigarette)	1700	410	270
Cigarettes-F (ng/cigarette)	150	190	150

NF, cigarette without filter tip; F, cigarette with filter tip

Table 5. Estimated exposure of United States residents to nitrosamines (National Research Council 1981)

Souce of exposure	Nitrosamines	Primary exposure route	Daily intake (μg/person)	
Beer	NDMA	Ingestion	0.34	
Cosmetics	NDELA	Dermal absorption	0.41	
Cooked meat, cooked bacon	NPYR	Ingestion	0.17	
Scotch whiskey	NDMA	Ingestion	0.03	
Cigarette smoking	VNA[a]	Inhalation	0.3	
	NDELA	Inhalation	0.5	
	NNN	Inhalation	6.1	16.2[c]
	NNK	Inhalation	2.9	
	NAT + NAB	Inhalation	7.2	
Snuff dipping	VNA[a]	Ingestion	3.1	
	NDELA	Ingestion	6.6	
	NNN	Ingestion	75.0	170.5[c]
	NNK	Ingestion	16.1	
	NAT + NAB	Ingestion	73.4	
	Iso-NNAL[b]	Ingestion	6.0	

[a] Brunnemann et al. 1982; average values from the leading five US fine-cut tobaccos used for snuff dipping in 1981; assumed consumption, 10 g/day; VNA = NDMA + NPYR + NMOR
[b] Brunnemann et al. (1987; in press)
[c] Sum of tobacco-specific nitrosamines

NDMA, nitrosodimethylamine; NDELA, nitrosodiethanolamine; NPYR, nitrosopyrrolidine; VNA, volatile nitrosamines; NNN, NNK, NAT, NAB, Red NNA see footnotes Table 3 concentrations of nitrosamines found in any other consumer product. This applies especially to snuff brands in the USA. In 1981, the US National Academy of Sciences compared the estimated exposure of US residents to nitrosamines (Table 5). We have amended this table to include the daily exposure of an "average snuff-dipper" to nitrosamines (National Research Council 1981; Hoffmann et al. 1986). These data document the fact that, on a daily basis, it is the tobacco consumer who is exposed to the highest amounts of carcinogenic N-nitrosamines, disregarding exposures in a few occupational settings (Preussmann, this volume).

Furthermore, as will be discussed later, it is also likely that nicotine is endogenously N-nitrosated. The resulting nitrosamines add to the body burden of TSNA for the tobacco consumer. For example, in cigarette smokers we found nicotine in higher concentrations in cervical mucus than in serum (Sasson et al. 1985). One may thus hypothesize that NNN and NNK may be formed in cervical fluids, and we are currently exploring this phenomenon analytically. Other factors which may contribute to the increased rate of cervix cancer in cigarette smokers are infections by human papilloma virus (zur Hausen, this volume) and mutagens in the mucus (Holly et al. 1986).

Biochemistry of TSNA

The high concentration of the nitrosamines derived from the *Nicotiana* alkaloids in tobacco products, their tobacco specificity, and their high carcinogenic activity required studies on their biochemical effects in mammalian systems (Hecht et al. 1983; Hoffmann and Hecht 1985).

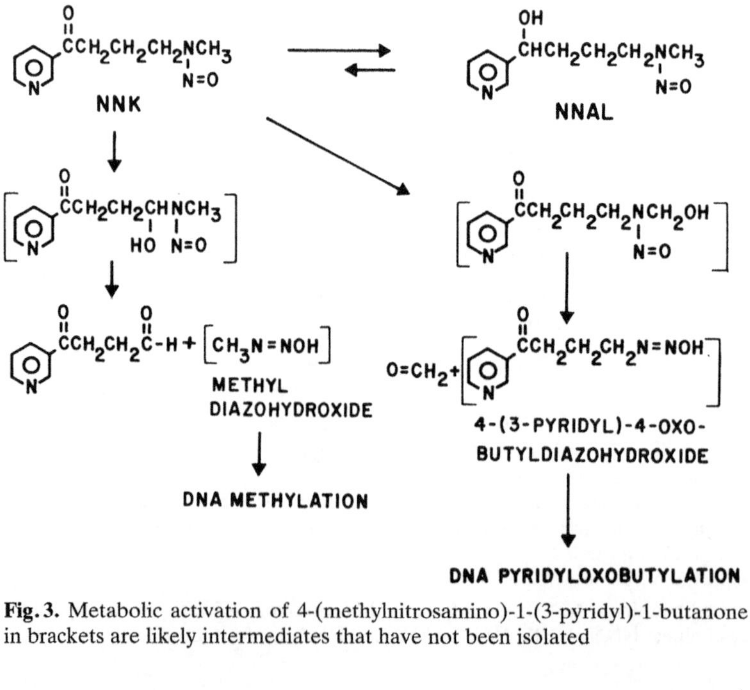

Fig. 3. Metabolic activation of 4-(methylnitrosamino)-1-(3-pyridyl)-1-butanone (NNK). Structures in brackets are likely intermediates that have not been isolated

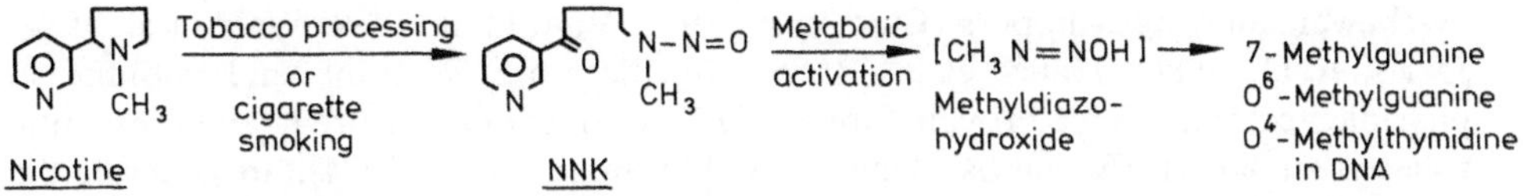

Fig. 4. Scheme linking nicotine to formation of the promutagenic DNA adducts, O^6-methylguanine and O^4-methylthymidine

Figure 3 summarizes the α-hydroxylation of NNK in vitro in animal and human tissues and in vivo in mice, rats, and hamsters. α-Hydroxylation of this unsymmetrical dialkylnitrosamine leads to two highly unstable α-hydroxynitrosamines. These decompose with formation of 4-(3-pyridyl)-4-oxobutanal and formaldehyde as well as two unstable diazohydroxides, namely, methyl diazohydroxide and 4-(3-pyridyl)-4-oxobutyldiazohydroxide. Methyldiazohydroxide is a known methylating agent. When rats were treated with NNK, 7-methylguanine, O^6-methylguanine, and O^4-methylthymidine were formed in the DNA of lung, liver, and nasal mucosa (Castonguay et al. 1984; Hecht et al. 1986; Belinsky et al. 1986). All of these are organs in which NNK induces tumors. Studies with cultured human buccal mucosa, trachea, esophagus, bronchus, peripheral lung, and bladder have shown that these tissues, too, can metabolize NNK by α-hydroxylation (Castonguay et al. 1983). Therefore, it is reasonable to expect that snuff-dipping and smoking will lead to formation of methylated bases in the DNA of oral or bronchial tissues of tobacco users. O^6-Methylguanine and O^4-methylthymidine have been shown to cause miscoding of DNA and are important in regard to tumor initiation. Figure 4 presents a scheme showing the link of the major and habituating tobacco alkaloid, nicotine, with the promutagenic DNA adduct O^6-methylguanine, and O^4-methylthymidine.

As was discussed, the α-hydroxylation of NNK at the N-methyl group leads to the alkylating agent 4-(3-pyridyl)-4-oxobutyldiazohydroxide. The same intermediate is formed upon α-hydroxylation of NNN (Hoffmann and Hecht 1985). We are currently exploring the DNA adduct(s) of this alkylating metabolite in vitro and in vivo. The isolation of such DNA adduct(s) will be of major significance because of the specificity of their origin from tobacco. After all, they derive strictly from nicotine *via* tobacco specific N-nitrosamines.

The possibility that reactive metabolites of NNK form adducts with globin is of considerable interest. Upon hydrolysis of such adducts, the released metabolite could be quantitatively determined in human blood either by radioimmunoassay or by postlabeling. This could be a suitable biological marker for measuring the uptake and possibly also the endogenous formation of tobacco-specific carcinogens as a result of tobacco use or environmental exposure to tobacco smoke.

Biological Markers

Currently, exhaled carbon monoxide, carboxyhemoglobin, thiocyanate, and/or nicotine as well as its major metabolite cotinine measured in saliva, serum, and/or urine serve as indicators for the uptake of tobacco smoke by smokers. Nicotine and cotinine are also quantitated as indicators for the absorption of tobacco constituents by chewers and snuff-dippers (Butts et al. 1974; Vogt et al. 1979; Wald et al. 1984; Jarvis et al. 1984; Haley et al. 1985). Furthermore, nicotine and cotinine in physiological fluids have proven to be useful indicators of exposure to environmental tobacco smoke (ETS; Jarvis et al. 1984; Hoffmann et al. 1984). In general, the amount of nicotine and its metabolites in blood and urine of nonsmokers exposed to ETS corresponds to no more than a few percent of the levels measured in a 20-cigarettes-a-day smoker. However, the comparison of the uptake of nicotine by active smokers and by involuntary smokers, as measured in physiological fluids, can be misleading. First, in mainstream smoke, nicotine is present in the particulate phase, but in ETS it is predominately in the vapor phase (Eudy et al. 1985). Second, the elimination times for cotinine in passive smokers are significantly slower than those in active smokers. In plasma of the active smoker, elimination of cotinine takes 18.5 (15.6–27.8) h and, in plasma of passive smokers, 49.7 (45–60) h; in urine it is 21.9 (12.6–31.6) h and 32.7 (23.9–42.6) h, respectively (Sepkovic and Haley 1985).

As discussed earlier, the measurement of nicotine and cotinine does not reflect the uptake of tobacco carcinogens per se. As discussed previously, it is possible that nicotine and the other tobacco alkaloids are precursors to endogenously formed TSNA. For the time being, this has only been demonstrated indirectly in that four studies have clearly shown increased urinary excretion of nitrosoproline and nitrosothioproline in the urine of cigarette smokers. This means that smokers have a significantly higher potential for endogenous nitrosamine formation than nonsmokers (Hoffmann and Brunnemann 1983; Ladd et al. 1984; Tsuda et al. 1986; Lu et al. 1986). We are now determining the endogenous formation of TSNA in tobacco users as well as means to inhibit the in vivo formation of TSNA.

In these assays, as well as in past studies on the reduction of tobacco smoke constituents, we are primarily interested in the mechanisms leading to a reduction of carcinogens during the processing or smoking of tobacco products, or in those leading to an inhibition of the endogenous formation in subjects who are voluntarily or involuntarily exposed to tobacco-derived materials. We realize that the reduction of tumorigenic agents and carcinogens in tobacco products can be of some benefit to those continuously exposed to these agents, but we continue to emphasize that only abstinence assures a major reduction of risk for those diseases associated with the exposure to tobacco and tobacco smoke.

Perspectives

One does not have to understand all of the factors involved in tobacco toxicology and tobacco carcinogenesis in order to eliminate the known or suspected risk factors associated with the exposure to tobacco products. In fact, we advocate abstention from tobacco use. However, we realize that the human dependency on tobacco will not disappear in the near future. The continuing numerical rise in cancer cases among cigarette smokers in many developed countries is not encouraging. Thus, it must be the goal of laboratory studies to strengthen the epidemiological evidence on the association between the various forms of cancer and exposure to tobacco and/or tobacco smoke.

Epidemiological methods may never be sensitive enough to establish a low risk factor for involuntary smoking with sufficient significance. We are confident that biochemical data will clarify some of the current uncertainties in respect to passive smoking and an increased risk for cancer. Such data will include the measurement of the absorption of tobacco carcinogens, their retention and activation to reactive species by nonsmokers as well as knowledge on the repair of the miscoding properties induced in DNA by tobacco constituents. In recent years, highly sensitive analytical and biochemical methods have been developed. Their application to tobacco carcinogenesis will provide the answers to many of the remaining questions. The newly emerging laboratory data in tobacco carcinogenesis will also contribute to a better understanding of chemical carcinogenesis. For example, they have given new directives for an understanding of the causal association between betel quid chewing and oral cancer. Furthermore, the data on tobacco-specific carcinogens have strengthened the evidence that nitrosamines are indeed human carcinogens. The utilization of biological markers in estimating tobacco exposure has greatly stimulated the concept of biological markers in occupational and environmental toxicology. Tobacco carcinogenesis will certainly also be greatly enhanced by the progress in chemical carcinogenesis. Interrelated studies will hopefully elucidate the many remaining challenges in tobacco carcinogenesis and contribute to the reduction of risk of all tobacco-related cancers.

Acknowledgements. We appreciate the editorial assistance of Mrs. Ilse Hoffmann and Mrs. Bertha Stadler.

References

Belinsky SA, White CM, Boucheron JA, Richardson FC, Swenberg JA, Anderson M (1986) Accumulation and persistence of DNA adducts in respiratory tissue of rats following multiple administration of the tobacco-specific carcinogen 4-(N-methyl-N-nitrosamino)-1-(3-pyridyl)-1-butanone. Cancer Res 46:1280–1284

Bernfeld P, Homburger F, Russfield AB (1974) Strain differences in the response of inbred Syrian hamsters to cigarette smoke inhalation. JNCI 53:1141–1157

Bock FG, Swain AP, Stedman RL (1971) Composition studies on tobacco LXIV. Tumor-promoting activity of subfractions of the weak acid fraction of cigarette smoke condensate. JNCI 47:429–436

Brunnemann KD, Scott JC, Hoffmann D (1982) N-nitrosomorpholine and other volatile N-nitrosamines in snuff tobacco. Carcinogenesis 3:693–696

Brunnemann KD, Genoble L, Hoffmann D (1987) Identification and analysis of a new tobacco-specific N-nitrosamine, 4-(methylnitrosamino)-4-(3-pyridyl)-1-butanol. Carcinogenesis 8 (in press)

Butts WC, Kuehneman M, Widdowson GM (1974) Automated method for determining serum thiocyanate to distinguish smokers from nonsmokers. Clin Chem 20:1344–1348

Castonguay A, Stoner GD, Schut HAJ, Hecht SS (1983) Metabolism of tobacco-specific N-nitrosamines by cultured human tissues. Proc Natl Acad Sci USA 80:6694–6697

Castonguay A, Tharp R, Hecht SS (1984) Kinetics of DNA methylation of the tobacco specific carcinogen 5-(methyl-nitrosamino)-1-(3-pyridyl)-1-butanone in F344 rats. IARC Sci Publ 57:805–810

Dalbey WE, Nettesheim P, Griesemer R, Caton JE, Guerin MR (1980) Chronic inhalation of cigarette smoke by F344 rats. JNCI 64:383–388

Doll R (1971) Cancers related to smoking. Proceedings of the 2nd world conference on smoking and health. Pitman Medical, London, pp 10–23

Doll R, Hill AB (1950) Smoking and carcinoma of the lung. Preliminary report. Br Med J 2:739–748
Dontenwill WP (1974) Tumorigenic effect of chronic cigarette smoke inhalation on Syrian golden hamsters. In: Karbe E, Park JF (eds) Experimental lung cancer. Carcinogenesis and bioassays. Springer, Berlin Heidelberg New York, pp 331–359
Dontenwill W, Chevalier HJ, Harke HP, Lafrenz U, Reckzeh G, Schneider B (1973) Investigations on the effects of chronic cigarette smoke inhalation in Syrian golden hamsters. JNCI 51:1781–1832
Dontenwill W, Chevalier HJ, Harke HP, Klimisch HJ, Reckzeh G, Fleischmann B, Keller W (1977) Experimentelle Untersuchungen über die tumorerzeugende Wirkung von Zigarettenrauch-Kondensaten an der Mäusehaut, VII. Mitteilung. Einzelbefunde von Kondensaten verschiedener modifizierter Zigaretten. Z Krebsforsch 89:145–151
Eudy LW, Thorne FA, Heavor DL, Green CR, Ingebrethsen BJ (1985) Studies on vapor-particulate phase distribution of environmental nicotine by selected trapping and detection methods. 39th Tobacco Chemists Research Conference, Montreal, Canada, abstract, p 25
Haley NJ, Sepkovic DW, Hoffmann D, Wynder EL (1985) Cigarette smoking as a risk for cardiovascular disease, part VI. Compensation with nicotine availability as a single variable. Clin Pharmacol Ther 38:164–170
Hecht SS, Thorne RL, Maronpot RR, Hoffmann D (1975) A study of tobacco carcinogenesis XIII. Tumor-promoting subfractions of the weakly acidic fraction. JNCI 55:1329–1336
Hecht SS, Carmella S, Mori H, Hoffmann D (1981) A study of tobacco carcinogenesis XX. Role of catechol as major cocarcinogen in the weakly acidic fraction of smoke condensate. JNCI 66: 163–169
Hecht SS, Castonguay A, Rivenson A, Mu B, Hoffmann D (1983) Tobacco specific nitrosamines: carcinogenicity, metabolism and possible role in human cancer. J Environ Sci Health [C] 1:1–54
Hecht SS, Trushin N, Castonguay A, Rivenson A (1986) A study of chemical carcinogenesis 88. Comparative carcinogenicity and DNA methylation in F344 rats by 4-(methylnitrosamino)-1-(3-pyridyl)-1-butanone and N-nitrosodimethylamine. Cancer 46:498–502
Herning RI, Jones RT, Bachman J, Mines AH (1981) Puff volume increases when low-nicotine cigarettes are smoked. Br Med J 283:187–189
Hoffmann D, Brunnemann KD (1983) Endogenous formation of N-nitrosoproline in cigarette smokers. Cancer Res 43:5570–5574
Hoffmann D, Hecht SS (1985) Perspectives in cancer research. Nicotine-derived N-nitrosamines and tobacco-related cancer: current status and future directions. Cancer Res 45:935–944
Hoffmann D, Wynder EL (1971) A study of tobacco carcinogenesis XI. Tumor initiators, tumor accelerators, and tumor promoting activity of condensate fractions. Cancer 27:848–864
Hoffmann D, Wynder EL (1972) Selective reduction of tumorigenicity of tobacco smoke II. Experimental approaches. JNCI 48:1855–1868
Hoffmann D, Wynder EL (1986) A study of tobacco carcinogenesis XXX. Chemical constituents and bioactivity of tobacco smoke. In: Zaridze DG, Peto R (eds) A Major International Health Hazard. IARC Sci Publ 74 (in press)
Hoffmann D, Tso TC, Gori GB (1980) The less harmful cigarette. Prev Med 9:287–296
Hoffmann D, Haley NJ, Adams JD, Brunnemann KD (1984) Tobacco sidestream smoke: uptake by nonsmokers. Prev Med 13:608–617
Hoffmann D, Harley NH, Fisenne I, Adams JD, Brunnemann KD (1986) Carcinogenic agents in snuff. JNCI 76:435–437
Holly EA, Petrakis NL, Friend NF, Sarles DL, Lee RE, Flander LD (1986) Mutagenic mucus in the cervix of smokers. JNCI 76:983–986
IARC: International Agency for Research on Cancer (1985) Tobacco habits other than smoking; betel-quid and areca-nut chewing; and some related nitrosamines. IARC, Lyon, France (Monograph No 37)
IARC: International Agency for Research on Cancer (1986) Tobacco smoking. IARC, Lyon, France (Monograph No 38)
Jarvis MJ, Tunstall-Pedoe H, Feyerabend C, Vesley C, Salvojee Y (1984) Biochemical markers of smoke absorption and self-reported exposure to passive smoking. J Epidemiol Commun Health 38:335–339
Ladd KF, Newmark HL, Archer MC (1984) N-Nitrosation of proline in smokers and nonsmokers. JNCI 73:83–87

LaVoie EL, Shigematsu A, Tucciarone PL, Adams JD, Hoffmann D (1985) Comparison of the steam-volatile components in commercial cigarette, pipe, and chewing tobaccos. J Agric Food Chem 33:547–552
Leuchtenberger C, Leuchtenberger R (1970) Effects of chronic inhalation of whole fresh cigarette smoke and of its gas phase on pulmonary tumorigenesis in Snell's mice. In: Nettesheim P, Hanna MG Jr, Daatherage JW Jr (eds) Morphology of experimental respiratory carcinogenesis. US AEC, Oak Ridge, TN, pp 329–346
Levin ML, Goldstein H, Gerhardt PR (1950) Cancer and tobacco smoking. A preliminary report. JAMA 143:336–338
Lu SH, Ohshima H, Fu HM, Tian Y, Li FM, Blettner M, Wahrendorf J, Bartsch H (1986) Urinary excretion of N-nitrosamino acids and nitrate by inhabitants of high- and low-risk areas for esophageal cancer in Northern China: endogenous formation of nitrosoproline and its inhibition by vitamin C. Cancer Res 46:1485–1491
Mohr U, Reznik G (1978) Tobacco carcinogenesis. In: Harris CC (ed) Pathogenesis and therapy of lung cancer. Dekker, New York, pp 263–367
Mueller FH (1939) Tabakmissbrauch und Lungencarcinom. Z Krebsforsch 49:57–84
National Research Council (1981) The health effects of nitrate, nitrite and N-nitroso compounds. National Academy Press, Washington, DC, p 51
Royal College of Physicians (1983) Health or smoking? Follow-up report of the Royal College of Physicians. Pitman, London
Sasson IM, Haley NJ, Hoffmann D, Wynder EL, Hellberg D, Nilsson S (1985) Cervical neoplasia and cigarette smoking: quantitation of smoke constituents in cervical mucus. New Engl J Med 312:315–316
Schairer E, Schoeninger E (1943) Lungenkrebs and Tabakverbrauch. Z Krebsforsch 54:261–269
Sepkovic DW, Haley NJ (1986) Metabolism of nicotine in smokers and nonsmokers. In: William RM et al (eds) Physiology and pharmacology of nicotine. Plenum, New York (in press)
Tsuda M, Nutsuma J, Sato S, Hirayama T, Kakizoe T, Sugimura T (1986) Increase in the levels of N-nitrosoproline, N-nitrosothioproline, and N-nitroso-2-methylthioproline in human urine by cigarette smoking. Cancer Lett 30:117–124
US Surgeon General (1982) The health consequences of smoking: cancer US Public Health Service, DHHS publication No (PHS) 82–50179
US Surgeon General (1983) The health consequences of smoking: cardiovascular disease. US Public Health Service, DHHS publication No (PHS) 84-50204
US Surgeon General (1986) Report of the surgeon general's advisory committee on the health consequences of using smokeless tobacco. Washington, DC, NIH Publ No 862874
Van Duuren BL, Goldschmidt BM (1976) Cocarcinogenic and tumor promoting agents in tobacco carcinogenesis. JNCI 56:1237–1242
Vogt TM, Selvin S, Billings JH (1979) Smoking cessation program: baseline carbon monoxide and serum thiocyanate levels as predictors of outcome. Am J Publ Health 69:1156–1159
Wald NJ, Boreham J, Bailey A, Ritchie C, Haddow JE, Knight G (1984) Urinary cotinine as marker for breathing other people's tobacco smoke. Lancet 1:230–231
Wynder EL, Graham EA (1950) Tobacco smoking as a possible etiological factor in bronchiogenic carcinoma. A study of six hundred and eighty-four proven cases. JAMA 143:329–336
Wynder EL, Hoffmann D (1961) Present status of laboratory studies on tobacco carcinogenesis. Acta Pathol Microbiol Scand 52:110–132
Wynder EL, Hoffmann D (1967) Tobacco and tobacco smoke. Studies in experimental carcinogenesis. Academic, New York

Primary Prevention of Tobacco-Related Cancer*

E. L. WYNDER and M. A. ORLANDI

Introduction

For more than a century, tobacco usage has been shown to induce cancer in man. As early as 1795, Soemmering described a cancer of the lip induced by pipe smoking. However, it was not until the twentieth century that the enormous rise in lung cancer elicited serious interest as a tobacco-related problem. As we reflect upon this history, we need to appreciate that a monograph on lung cancer written by Adler in 1912 included the question: "Is it worthwhile to write on such a rare disease?" Even in 1939, when Mueller in Germany had reported on the increased risk of lung cancer in smokers, the admission of a lung cancer patient to Barnes Hospital in St. Louis, Missouri, prompted the staff to call interns and residents together to see such a rare case (Mueller 1939). In 1950, when the first major papers on the role of tobacco in the etiology of lung cancer were published, lung cancer had become a common observation in men though still relatively uncommon in women (Doll and Hill 1950; Levin et al. 1950; Wynder and Graham 1950). Today, in most developed countries, lung cancer is the most common cause of cancer deaths in males and is readily on its way to becoming the leading cause of cancer deaths in women by the end of this decade (International Agency for Research on Cancer 1986). The retrospective studies of 1950 were followed by a series of prospective studies, all showing an increase in lung cancer proportional to the number of cigarettes smoked and the duration of the habit.

But it was not until 1962 that a committee of the British Royal College of Physicians and not until 1964 that the US Surgeon General's Advisory Committee on Smoking and Health (US Department of Health, Education, and Welfare 1964) determined that cigarette smoking was causally associated with lung cancer, a conclusion since amply confirmed not only in epidemiological studies, but by biological and chemical investigations as well (Wynder and Hoffmann 1967; Mohr and Reznik 1978).

Both retrospective and prospective studies also showed a causal relationship of tobacco use to cancer of the mouth, larynx, esophagus, bladder, and pancreas (US Department of Health and Human Services 1982; International Agency for Research on Cancer 1986).

Unlike the urgent responses to epidemics of infectious diseases for which history provides many examples, there is a remarkable reluctance to take preventive action in the face of the risk for the chronic yet devastating illnesses associated with tobacco

* Supported by U.S. National Cancer Institute grants no. PO1-CA-32167, CA-17613, CA-38219, and CA-41621

smoking. In the case of the established causal relationship of smoking to lung cancer this reluctance is especially astonishing in view of the magnitude of this cancer problem. As we debate how to reduce tobacco-related cancers, we need to examine the obstacles to prevention efforts which account for the reluctance to act forcefully.

Obstacles to Primary Prevention of Tobacco-Related-Cancer

Medical Community

If physicians became more actively involved in health promotion rather than limiting their practice to the care and treatment of patients, there would surely be fewer smokers today. Yet, the majority of physicians are not prevention-oriented nor are the hospitals.

Although physicians as a group have given up smoking more readily than their patients have (Doll and Peto 1976, 1977), public health authorities and medical associations are only now beginning to be adamant about the goal of a smoking-free society by the turn of the millenium (DeVita 1983; American Medical Association 1986). The lateness of these efforts makes them no less urgent when we face the reality of an estimated 130000 deaths from lung cancer and 146000 new cases of lung cancer as statistics for 1986 in the USA alone – not even considering other tobacco-related cancers (American Cancer Society 1986).

Individual

It is probably within the nature of man to deny or ignore a risk inherent in a self-imposed behavior. Even when the risk is acknowledged, we find it difficult to sacrifice momentary pleasure for a promised distant health benefit. This may in part be due to an illusion of immortality which we like to nurture in view of our inability to accept the reality of death. Moreover, some of us may, in fact, suffer from a subconscious death wish leading us to challenge fate by engaging in risk-taking behavior, a phenomenon frequently seen among young people (American Health Foundation 1976).

Thus, a key obstacle to disease prevention in general and to cessation of tobacco use in particular is human nature. While we tend to protest in large groups against pollution of our forests and rivers, against additives in food, and certainly against nuclear dangers, we ignore the importance of our individual behavior in terms of what we smoke, eat, and drink. The difficulties in any individual effort to avoid the risks associated with tobacco use are compounded by the fact that tobacco use creates pharmacologically based dependence (National Institute on Drug Abuse 1979).

Society

The vested interests in tobacco products of certain segments of society are obvious obstacles to programs directed to reduce if not eliminate tobacco use. This includes the tobacco industry from the farmer to the manufacturer and distributor of tobacco products, to the vast commercial interests including television, radio, print media, advertising, and public relations companies involved in the marketing of such products. Dependence of governmental programs on tax revenues from the foregoing activities and pressure from those regions or segments of the country that derive significant income from tobacco add to the weight of importance of the tobacco economy. It is said that "politics is the art of the possible." Some aspects relating to the politics of antitobacco programs are and some are not possible to circumvent. It is clear, for the stated reasons, that society as a whole represents a key obstacle to prevention of chronic diseases associated with tobacco use.

Opportunities to Reduce Tobacco-Related Diseases

Successful strategies for reducing and eventually eliminating tobacco-related diseases require the contributions of various segments of our society. We will discuss such strategies in increasing order of their importance.

The Low-Yield Cigarette

We are often asked why those in academic research should work on the chemistry and biology of tobacco and tobacco smoking with a view to reducing toxic and tumorigenic constituents. As long as we, as a society, condone the manufacture of tobacco products, they will be tried by consumers and, because of an apparent satisfaction or pharmacologic dependence that lies in the use of tobacco products, these will continue to be used. It is particularly difficult to reach developing societies and, within developed countries, lower socioeconomic groups with health education efforts. Since we still have more than 55 million cigarette smokers in the USA, it behooves us to continue work in the area of "less harmful cigarettes," while always emphasizing that no cigarette can be safe. During the past four decades since we first produced skin cancer in experiments with "tar" applied to mice and rabbits, the tar yield in the smoke of cigarettes in most parts of the world has been dramatically reduced, with somewhat lesser reduction in nicotine (IARC 1986). Laboratory studies have shown lower tumorigenic activity of tar from low-yield cigarettes compared with the activities of tar obtained in the 1950s concomitant with a specific reduction in PAH and other tumorigenic components. It would appear, therefore, that a reduction in tumorigenic potency of smoke condensate per cigarette has taken place. Perhaps, this may explain why fewer bronchial changes were seen in human autopsy material among cigarette smokers in the 1970s as compared with the 1960s (Auerbach et al. 1980). More pertinent, of course, is whether the risk for various tobacco-related diseases among smokers of low-yield cigarettes has actually been lowered. Comparisons of lung cancer rates among long-term smokers of filter cigarettes with those of smokers who have only used nonfilter cigarettes appear to be in general agreement that there is a decline of about 20% in risk among those who have shifted to filter cigarettes for at least 10 years, while this decline approximates 50% for those who have smoked filter cigarettes only (Figs. 1 and 2). It is likely that these findings are due both to a reduction in tar exposure and a specific reduction of tumorigenic

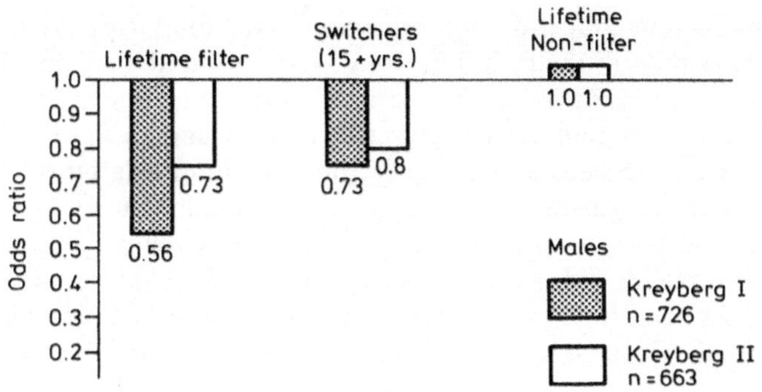

Fig. 1. Age-adjusted odds ratios for lung cancer in men for lifetime filter-cigarette smokers and long-term switchers (1st year) relative to lifetime smokers of nonfilter cigarettes. (Unpublished data from Wynder and Kabat 1986)

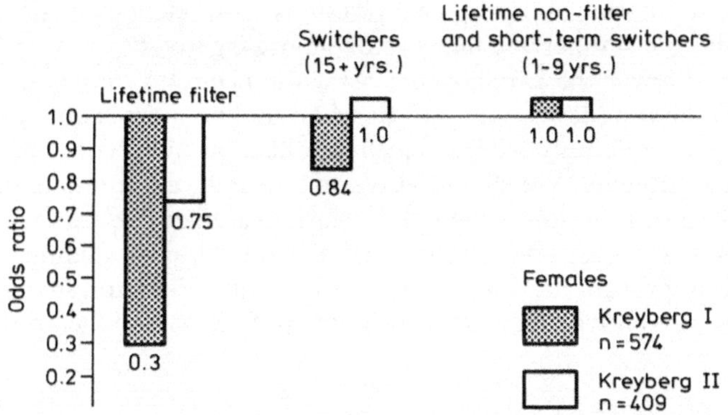

Fig. 2. Age-adjusted odds ratios for lung cancer in women for lifetime filter-cigarette smokers and long-term switchers (1st year) relative to smokers of nonfilter cigarettes and short-term switchers. (Unpublished data from Wynder and Kabat 1986)

potency of the smoke as compared with that from cigarettes smoked 30 years ago. It is noteworthy that there has been a shift in the ratio of squamous cell lung cancer to glandular types of cancer during the past four decades (Melamed et al. 1984; Dodds et al. 1986). This shift may, in part, relate to deeper inhalation of cigarette mainstream smoke as a consequence of the reduced delivery of tar and nicotine in the smoke of low-yield cigarettes.

Any consideration of risk reduction achieved by smoking a "less harmful cigarette" that may be valid with regard to lung cancer risk, may not apply to the risk for coronary heart disease (US Public Health Service 1983). To the extent that nicotine plays a role in respect to cardiovascular events, the reduction of nicotine delivery in the smoke of most low-yield cigarettes may not be sufficient to have a significant effect. Because coronary artery disease is a consequence of the "double jeopardy" of smoking and hyperlipidemia, a key preventive approach to heart attack (the leading cause of death in the Western world) should also center on the reduction of serum cholesterol levels. This is an effort which we pursue in various parts of the USA through mass screenings and health education. In proportion to the total population, we have today fewer smokers than in the past, but those who do smoke tend to be relatively heavy smokers, i.e., in order to reach a desired level of nicotine in their bloodstream, they smoke a greater number of cigarettes or they smoke more intensely. For these reasons, we propose that the average tar content of cigarettes be lowered to 10 mg by the end of the decade and that no cigarette should deliver more than 14 mg of tar. There has been a debate as to the optimal nicotine delivery in the smoke of such cigarettes. Low yields of tar yet moderate yields of nicotine appear to be practical recommendations even though there is evidence to suggest that nicotine as such may play a role in the carcinogenicity of tobacco smoke (Hoffmann and Hecht 1986).

Generally, smokers are likely to adjust smoking habits in such a way that a desired amount of nicotine is inhaled; only in the case of ultralow yields of nicotine ($\leq$0.5 mg/cigarette with standardized machine-smoking) is it impossible for the smoker to fully compensate for desired nicotine uptake (Haley et al. 1985). If the availability of the nicotine in the smoke of a given cigarette is insufficient even after adjusting smoking intensity, the smoker will likely smoke more cigarettes.

In summary, in order to lower the carcinogenic risk from cigarette smoking, a global strategy should aim the products yielding 10 mg of tar and no more than 1 mg of nicotine per cigarette and preferably having selective reduction of specific toxic and tumorigenic smoke constituents. We should also strive to reduce the intake of dietary fat by the population so as to lower the risk for cardiovascular disease especially among smokers. But we must reemphasize that the only way to eliminate tobacco-related diseases is to prevent the onset of the smoking habit. This too should be possible in the realm of preventive medicine, which, like politics, is also the art of the possible.

Smoking Cessation

Cigarette smoking is a behavior that is most difficult to change. Nevertheless, an estimated 33 million Americans have quit the habit between 1964 and 1982. The majority, in fact more than 90%, stopped smoking without the aid of a formal smoking cessation treatment (Fig. 3). Approximately 33% of the adult population in the United States now smoke and this is the lowest figure in recent years (US Public Health Service 1979; Harris 1983). The large numbers of exsmokers in our adult society, particularly among older and better educated men, testify to some success of health education efforts; such efforts must yet be stepped up to motivate women in all segments of society and both men and women in lower socioeconomic groups towards smoking cessation (Fig. 4). Thus, continuing efforts to promote smoking cessation are of paramount importance. Although the percentage of smokers among both men and women has declined, the overall decrease among women has been slower. Among younger women smoking prevalence has actually increased somewhat. Unless smoking prevalence among women decreases significantly, it is expected that their current lung cancer rate may double by 1990 (US National Cancer Institute 1986).

It is now well established that the risk of lung cancer among exsmokers depends on the amount of cigarettes smoked and the years of smoking. Clearly, the fewer cig-

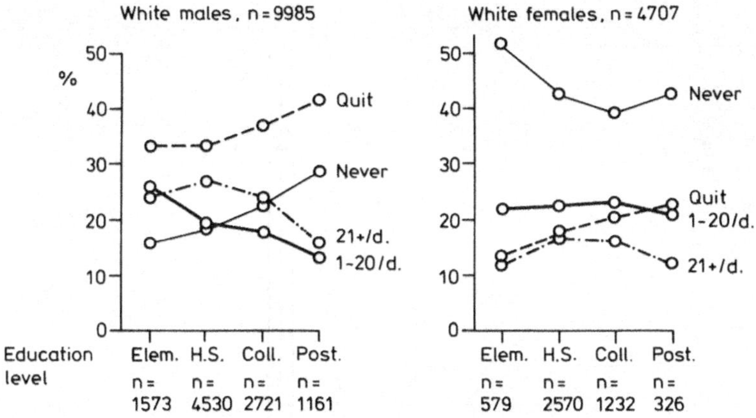

Fig. 3. Smoking by education

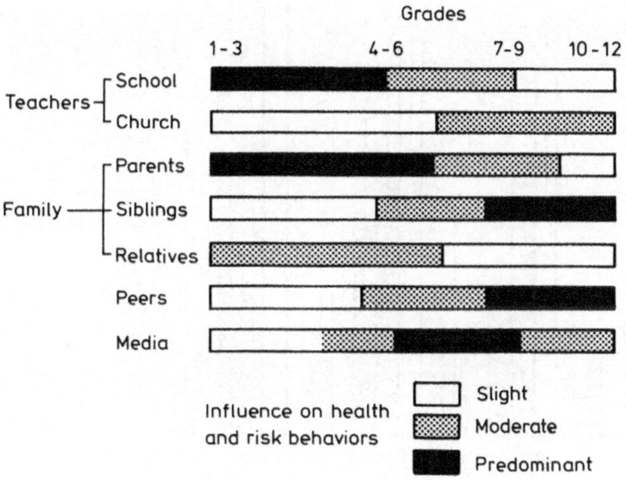

Fig. 4. Interpersonal dimensions of health promotion and education

arettes smoked per day and the shorter the history of smoking, the lower is the risk (Fig. 5). A variety of factors have been shown to be related to successful smoking cessation as described in the discussion which follows.

Difficulties of Quitting

Low self-esteem, the inherent illusion of immortality, low social class and, in women, the fear of weight gain as well as the pharmacologic dependence on tobacco smoking, are key variables responsible for failures of cessation attempts. Smoking habits are closely associated with occupational class and with ethnic and religious health traditions (Fig. 4).

There is overwhelming evidence that most who have given up smoking (about 95%) have done so on their own, while the other 5%, most of whom were heavy smokers required assistance.

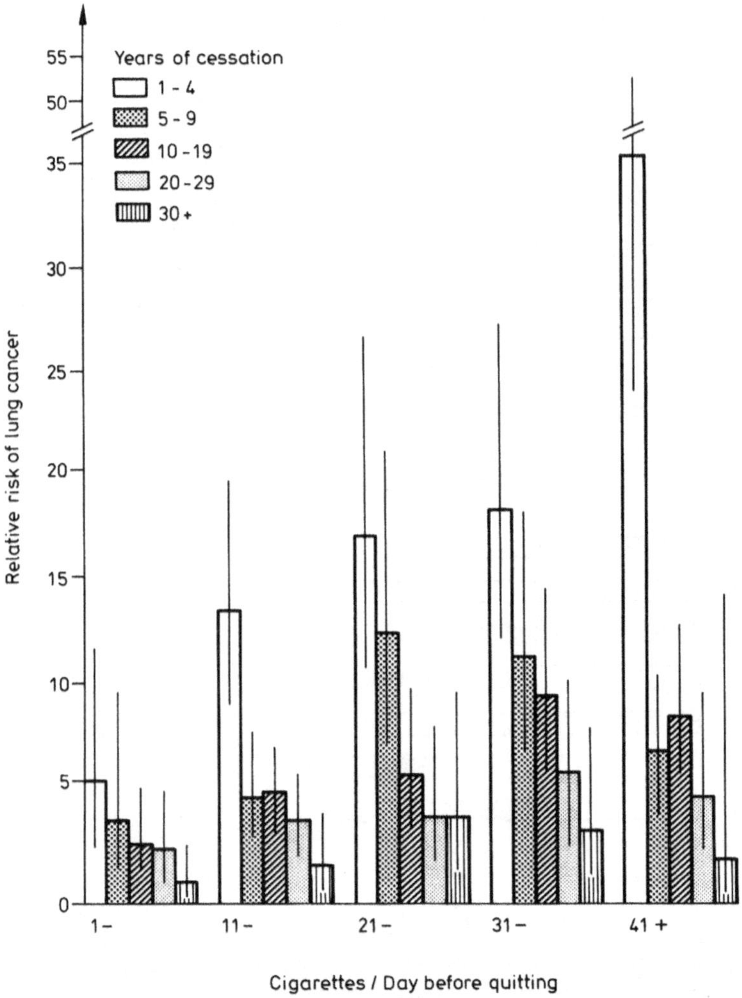

Fig. 5. Risk of lung cancer (and 95% confidence interval) by number of cigarettes smoked before quitting and years of cessation; males Kreyberg I and Kreyberg II

Antitobacco propaganda, peer pressure by both colleagues and family does work and social support is most important for the potential quitter. In the USA, our greatest concern is that there are still more than 55 million adult smokers. This sizable population group has become the target of a variety of public health interventions aimed at eliminating tobacco use.

Why is it so difficult for cigarette smokers to quit? The pharmacological objective of cigarette smoking is to deliver nicotine, a powerful primary reinforcer, to the nervous system. Smoking can deliver nicotine to the central nervous system within about 7 s and many smokers, particularly heavy smokers, have learned to adjust their smoking patterns in such a way that they are able to regulate their dosage of nicotine quite precisely (Gritz et al. 1976; Schachter 1978; Haley et al. 1985). Since smoking can be undertaken in a variety of circumstances and settings, these settings often become signals to smoke and as such they become incorporated as learned rewards for smoking. For example, learning that smoking a cigarette while drinking a beer is relaxing in a potentially stressful situation, is reinforcing. Once this is learned, it is possible for the situation itself to trigger the need for the cigarette.

The tenacity of the smoking habit is also upheld because of the many trials that occur during the course of a lifetime of a regular cigarette smoker. For example, 20 cigarettes per day adds up to more than 7000 cigarettes a year and each puff of a cigarette, is an occasion for experiencing one or more of the rewards that have become associated with cigarette smoking. There are few behaviors that can provide both psychological and pharmacological reinforcement at that rate of frequency.

On the other hand, the most powerful negative consequences of smoking relate to potential ill health effects at some point in the future. Thus, while the primary positive reinforcers for smoking are strong, immediate, and salient, the primary negative reinforcers are those factors that would work against the cigarette habit, tend to be weaker and less salient.

Interventions that have been developed in an attempt to eliminate tobacco use can be broken down into five general categories:

1. Public intervention campaigns: community-based or information-based campaigns
2. Self-help oriented programs
3. Structured group approaches or basic group support programs
4. Individualized behavioral intervention programs
5. Pharmacological interventions

Public Intervention Campaigns

Public intervention campaigns have evolved over the years reflecting the state-of-the-art of our understanding of the factors that contribute to smoking and of those that enable individuals to quit. Prior to the 1970s, public information programs or community-based programs tended to simply inform individuals about the danger of smoking. This was expected to motivate individuals to stop smoking. The information was provided through a variety of media and channels including pamphlets, books, and public service announcements on television and radio. By and large, this entire effort was referred to as an "information only" type of campaign. The lack of success of such programs engendered significant research to determine why the newly gained knowledge of the dangers of smoking did not cause an individual to quit. The answers to this question gave us new insights. First, behavior change results from a series of steps which usually, but not always, begin with changes in knowledge. Acceptance of knowledge as a directive to change behavior and complying with this particular directive is opposed by the belief that negative consequences of noncompliance would not actually befall one though the directive may be valid for others. Thus, in addition to accepting knowledge, an individual must be convinced about the relevance of the information to himself or herself. Further, a person's value system and attitudes towards health, or disease, a person's general attitude towards complacency with a status quo vs wanting an upward change, all of these factors tend to intervene with responses to directives for change that are based on knowledge alone.

The second recognition has to do with our understanding of a person's history of tobacco smoking. Whether a smoker is receptive to any particular message of intervention in behavior depends very much on the reason for smoking at the time the message is delivered. We can define four different categories of cigarette smokers. The first category consists of people who are just starting the habit. In the second category are persons who have gone beyond that initial experimentation phase and are now on their way to becoming habitual smokers. The third category is that of smokers who have decided to quit and are trying to do so. A fourth category are smokers who have quit, but have then decided to resume. These distinctions are important as factors which determine or predict the likelihood that a particular mode of intervention will be effective for them. Most intervention programs make no attempt to distinguish between individuals at these various stages in their history of smoking and herein lies one of the reasons why smoking cessation efforts are often judged to be relatively ineffective. The recognition of a need for interventions that address individuals at various stages in their personal history of smoking led to community-based studies such as the Stanford Three-Community and Five-Community Projects as well as the North Karelia Project (Vartianen et al. 1983) and others which have utilized televized smoking cessation techniques coupled with organized viewing groups (US Public Health Service 1984). In a collaborative group, individuals are encouraged to quit smoking, to join with other smokers who want to quit, and to watch a television program that is being broadcast publicly. This particular approach was designed to not only disseminate information about the dangers of smoking, but to also provide motivation to quit, to influence attitudes, value systems and beliefs, and to teach specific skills for quitting, all within the context of a supportive environment. Such approaches have tended to be far more effective than public information campaigns that focused on information alone.

Self-Help Oriented Programs

"Self-help" here is a bit of a misnomer. True self-help, i.e., quitting without help from any other individual or any other intervention program is what a vast majority of smokers provide for themselves. About 95% of all smokers who quit make the decision to quit and do so (US Public Health Service 1984). The study of individuals who have quit on their own has provided much insight into the factors which lead to successful quitting and has contributed to the development of therapeutic interventions for those individuals who have trouble quitting on their own. Such individuals may require assistance for self-help programs in the form of a booklet, a videotape, or a television program. In essence, quitting is done essentially away from direct contact with either a smoking cessation clinic or without the help of a particular therapist or counselor. This general approach tends to be highly cost-effective, even though the rates at which people quit with self-help oriented approaches are somewhat lower than the success rates in smoking cessation clinics (US Public Health Service 1984).

Structured Group Approach

This is the approach that many people consider when they think of smoking cessation programs. Clinic-based or structured group approaches grew directly out of the research that contributed to the development of more effective self-help approaches. In general, the clinic-based approach or the structured group approach is an opportunity for individuals interested in quitting but unable to do so on their own or with any form of self-help oriented approach. For such individuals, the structured group approach is often a viable alternative in that it allows them to engage in a learning process that will move them along, to the actual quitting as part of a supportive group, all of whom are smokers who reinforce each other's need and desire to quit. There is great emphasis on multiple components, providing the individual with a variety of skills and a variety of behavioral and cognitive strategies. There is definite orientation towards skills development, learning how to do something and then practicing it, for example, self-monitoring, keeping track of the number of cigarettes smoked during the day, recording the mood at the time each cigarette is smoked, and so forth. This form of self-awareness regarding the smoking habit tends to break down the major stimulus – response relationship and helps persons to recognize those stimuli that make them respond with smoking a cigarette. Monitoring of behavior and self-observation increases the self-awareness that helps to break down the undesirable responses to certain stimuli.

Individualized Behavior Intervention

An alternative to the clinic-based approach is the individual or face-to-face approach. In terms of cost-effectiveness, this could be viewed as one of the least useful approaches simply because it tends to engage one health professional and only one smoker during the course of the encounter. However, in general this intervention is very similar to that delivered through a structured group approach or through a self-help manual or a self-help television program, all of which would in the end be similar to the theoretical underpinnings of a state-of-the-art public information community-based campaign. The one difference is that the individual approach is often conducted by a trained psychotherapist or a psychiatrist and provides the opportunity for delving into issues of mental health that are unrelated to the smoking problem and would not be dealt with in the context of any of the other cessation methods. For instance, if an individual is smoking cigarettes because he/she is chronically depressed on account of a deep-seated mental health problem, it is less likely that such an individual will benefit directly from the learning of behavioral or cognitive skills that would be offered to them through the group approach or any of the other approaches described.

Pharmacological Approaches

Among pharmacological approaches to smoking cessation, the use of nicotine chewing gum is thought to hold promise particularly for heavy smokers due to its ability to minimize the withdrawal effects of nicotine while eliminating exposure to smoke

(Fagerstrom 1984). This should make it easier for an individual to quit and should enable heavy smokers to learn some of the behavioral skills that individuals who are less dependent on nicotine learn easily. Used properly, especially in conjunction with other smoking cessation methods, this can be a very good approach for controlling the urge to smoke for heavy smokers while they are in fact quitting and adopting some of the skills that will help them to maintain nonsmoking status. On the other hand, recent observations indicate that physicians should emphasize the need for gradual reduction of nicotine gum because of the possibility of sustained nicotine dependence with prolonged chewing of the gum (Hughes et al. 1986).

General Evaluation of Smoking Cessation Techniques

Several factors have made it difficult to interpret which of the intervention approaches have the greatest efficacy although data support the notion that smoking cessation approaches are generally effective. However, the percentage of smokers who benefit from these programs varies and is often in dispute. What is entirely unclear from most of the research, is which smokers benefit from which kinds of treatment. This confusion is due to the fact that few attempts have been made to study the efficacy of different smoking cessation techniques for subgroups of smokers. For example, desensitizing technique that make an individual feel more comfortable such as holding something like a cigarette in his hands may very well be most effective for those who smoke primarily to control anxiety, whereas aversive conditioning might be more appropriate for those who smoke primarily for positive reinforcement. Aversive conditioning utilizes changes in the way in which the cigarette smoke is inhaled, for example, holding the smoke in the lungs in such a way that it becomes physiologically aversive.

Most studies have not categorized different types of smokers, and have reported outcome measures as means for the group, thereby obscuring potentially significant variations among individuals. The fact that most of the methods utilize a multicomponent treatment approach, tends to compound the confusion. Further, when program success rates for any type of intervention approach are reported, the critical issue of adherence to the intervention protocols is seldom addressed.

In other words, many of those in a program who were counted as "successes" may not at all have used the techniques prescribed by the intervention. Despite this confusion, published research indicates that a participant in any such program has a 15%–20% chance of being abstinent after 1 year, with some programs reporting abstinence rates of 30% and 40%.

The histories of smoking cessation efforts have indicated that many quitters have often tried several different approaches before ultimately becoming successful.

Until we know more about the specific relationship between certain individual smokers and the quitting strategies most appropriate for them, a variety of approaches and program sites should be offered in any public policy that attempts to control smoking on a broad scale. In other words, no one approach tends to work for all individuals nor should any one approach be focused upon as the one public orientation towards smoking cessation for any geographic region or country because smokers cannot be viewed as a homogeneous group.

Special Opportunity for Smoking Cessation

One route of smoking control which unquestionably needs to be considered is the physician, as was shown by Russell et al. (1986), because most individuals tend to view the physician as a primary source of medical information. In an excellent position to provide both motivation and encouragement, the physician has the opportunity to promote a healthier lifestyle in a variety of ways. First, physicians should act as role models to their patients by not smoking. Further, physicians can provide the basic information that we were discussing, clarifying the specific risk associated with smoking, and the degree to which that risk can be reduced by smoking cessation or the decision not to smoke, which is most important for younger patients. Physicians can also encourage abstinence by giving direct advice and suggestions, taking their cue from a variety of available quit kits. They can make specific referrals for a patient to an ongoing structured smoking cessation program. They can also prescribe and monitor the use of specific cessation and maintenance strategies in their own office. If all physicians would give such advice to all of their patients, smoking in the population would be significantly reduced. Help should come from the medical profession, but is generally not available.

One of our staff members called 28 hospitals in the New York City area, posing as a smoker in need of help. Twenty-four had no service, one referred her to a hypnotist, and three referred her to clinics operated by the American Cancer Society. Clearly, in New York and in most other cities, smoking cessation clinics are not part of the vast outpatient service of hospitals. This medical oversight must be corrected. Both physicians and hospitals must take a more active role in smoking control if we are to reach the goal of a smoking-free healthier society.

For smoking cessation efforts at the work site we have trained nurses and nonmedical personnel, especially exsmokers to work with interested companies in providing smoking cessation courses that we have developed. Major corporations should have such a program available for their employees. The methods of smoking cessation include individual counseling, group counseling, hypnosis, acupuncture, and drugs like nicorette. These programs have a short-term success rate of around 50%, with a long-term success rate of 25%. The greatest success is in those who have been able to give up smoking before. Even a success rate of converting 25% to exsmokers is obviously desirable in both social and economic terms.

Legislation can also help by mandating taxes on tobacco products making it more difficult to purchase them, especially in large quantities.

The physician and a variety of organizations that can provide self-help oriented material should become active. Institutions that are ready, willing, and able to provide smoking cessation clinics should be promoted for individuals who need that form of structured help. The public media, including television and radio, should be utilized to the extent possible to promote nonsmoking by going beyond simply providing information and actually airing skills-development programs. Unions and trade organizations could help to institute work-site policies to help control smoking. Everything from outright no-smoking policies to a structured designation of limited smoking areas would be considered in this regard. Public places with policies for smoking control are powerful examples of a type of smoking control strategy.

Without doubt, making nonsmoking the social norm and providing the appropriate social support for smoking cessation will advance the goals of a smoking-free society and provide a healthier outlook for all people. To accomplish this, we as physicians, scientists, teachers, parents, relatives, societal leaders, colleagues, and friends can assist smokers to break the habit permanently. What is required of us, is our care and our committment.

Prevention of the Smoking Habit

Preferences for certain foods, exercise habits, a taste for tobacco and alcohol, habits of taking medication – all of these are established relatively early in life. A recent survey of male patients with lung cancer revealed that $\simeq 75\%$ of them had begun smoking cigarettes before they were 20 years old, the average age at onset being 17.4 years. Today's adolescents begin smoking even earlier. Among USA high school students who smoked on a regular basis, ⅔ began to do so in 9th grade when they were about 15 years old (US Department of Health and Human Services 1985).

It is clear that attempts to prevent the onset of smoking must be made as early in life as possible.

For our earliest health education we rely on the examples set and the teaching provided by parents and other family members. Studies have confirmed that the smoking habits of children are strongly correlated with those of their parents (Wohlford 1970; Borland and Rudolph 1975). We also have the opportunity to teach good health behavior through televized messages delivered by "spokesmen." The American Health Foundation, in collaboration with USA toymakers, has developed such characters and their messages which are being aired during children's programs. Whether these characters are on the side of the good or the bad habits is immediately known by their names: 4-U (For You) should become widely recognized as a self-respecting character and symbol of good health habits, his friend is U-4ia (Euphoria); "Fast-Lane' and "Couch Potato" are obviously on the other side of the issue. The topics of the health messages include cigarette smoking, smokeless tobacco, self-esteem, and the need for children to make their own and – hopefully the appropriate – health decisions.

The media have a very important role in delivering these educational messages as a motivating and compelling force. Success of such health education programs will depend on the quality, as well as on the intensity and duration, of their presentation.

In a more organized fashion, we can reach children in schools and in preschool programs. We are concerned about the lack of adequate school health education. In many countries, health education is a subject for which teachers are not trained, for which funds are not provided, and for which evaluation is not expected. Yet we ask, why should health education be treated differently from subjects like mathematics and history? They are all subjects that need to be learned. Many programs aimed at preventing the onset of the smoking habit in adolescents have shown short-term success (Botvin and Eng 1982; Flay 1985). However, they are usually based on a specific research protocol that did not have a long-term follow-up in respect to its efficacy as a smoking-prevention method.

A more comprehensive school-health education program developed by the American Health Foundation for use in the USA and internationally in several coun-

Table 1. Percentage of high school seniors who smoke ($n = 22000$). From Johnston et al. (1985)

	Males	Females
1975	26.9	26.4
1976	28.0	28.8
1977	27.1	30.0
1978	26.0	28.3
1979	22.3	27.8
1980	18.5	23.5
1981	18.1	21.7
1982	18.2	23.2
1983	19.2	22.2
1984	16.0	20.5

tries is the "Know Your Body (KYB) Program" (Williams et al. 1979). This multicomponent, teacher-delivered health promotion curriculum is designed to provide students in grades 1–9 with the basis for lifelong positive health decisions. Because health behavior is determined by a complex interaction of knowledge, attitudes, social influences, life experiences, and peer behavior, the KYB program incorporates life skills and decision-making modules in addition to an extensive information component. By fostering positive nutrition and exercise habits and discouraging use of tobacco, alcohol, and drugs among children, the program can significantly reduce the risk for cancer and heart disease as well as other life-threatening illnesses later in life.

An essential component of the KYB program is the annual biomedical screening. Students' height, weight, blood pressure, serum cholesterol, and fitness levels are assessed. The results from the screening are sent home to parents in an easily understood format which includes tips for reducing risk in areas where their child may have been deficient. Students are asked to record the results of their screening in their personal "health passport." This helps to make them aware of their health status, to personalize the program, and to highlight possible areas of intervention. Already by age 9, more than 40% of the children tested had one or more risk factor for cardiovascular diseases. The program, in respect to smoking, comes at a time when there is an overall decline in cigarette smoking among adolescents although not among girls (Table 1). Since female high school seniors now do more regular smoking than males, greater educational efforts must be directed towards women. Of particular concern is the fact that among high school students who do not plan to go to college, there are more who regularly smoke half a pack per day (20%) than among those who are college-bound (7.5%; Walter et al. 1985). Thus, in adolescence or adulthood, smoking, especially among men, is related to socioeconomic levels.

Strategies for Behavior Modification

The concept that the dose makes the therapy does not only apply to the treatment of disease, but applies equally to preventive medicine and, as part of this, to health education. Providing an insufficient dose of knowledge and behavior messages may not succeed in changing the health behavior of an individual. Health education means more than providing information. Our strategy, therefore, must be to provide the dose that has the chance to positively influence behavior. Foremost is the need for involvement of the students in planning health promotion. For instance, student workshops discuss tobacco advertising strategies. Models are used to demonstrate the impact of smoke on the body, while role playing teaches children to say no to tobacco offered by friends. To provide another example: children found to have cholesterol levels of about 170 mg% were invited to participate in a series of workshops; they were taught to lower their intake of saturated fat and cholesterol, to increase their intake of fiber and fish, to step-up their exercise program, and to keep food diaries. The mean cholesterol level of these children in October 1985 was 193 mg%, by April 1986 it was 179.9 mg%, a drop of 6.3%. We hope that repeated exposure to the concepts of KYB over 6 years of elementary school instruction will make this reduction even more dramatic and enduring. Intervention aimed at children as a group, be it in prevention of smoking, lowering of cholesterol, or reducing obesity, can be most cost-effective, particularly for high-risk individuals.

With the help of the nutrition department of the school system of the City of New York, we were able to give children greater choices in the cafeteria. Within a 2-week-period, a campaign directed at the increased use of skim milk brought a tenfold increase of the amount of low-fat milk being consumed. Other changes that we introduced into the cafeteria included a greater emphasis on fruit, vegetables, whole wheat bread, and a decreased consumption of red meat. As part of this effort, students were taught how to read food labels, especially paying attention to the lack of nutritional value in some snack foods and the excessive caloric and fat content of ice cream.

Periodic KYB newsletters, which children took home, informed their parents about what the children were taught in the school setting and also suggested changes in the home in support of the KYB concept. For instance, one newsletter contained a family contract to increase family consumption of complex carbohydrates. Parents also received a completed Health Passport with their children's screening results. The majority of the parents found the screening useful.

The success of the program depends on the participation of a KYB coordinator, the involvement of the teachers, parents, students, and community, and on the quality, intensity, and duration of the effort.

Studies have shown that antismoking programs, initiated after the age of 12 (seventh grade) may be too late. The best time to begin health education is probably in kindergarten or grade 1. In the early grades, children are most impressionable and perhaps most likely to learn how to avoid substance abuse. The fact that we find changes in weight, blood pressure, and serum cholesterol, all related to changes in behavior as a consequence of intervention programs, suggests that positive health habits can be developed and also bodes well for decreased smoking rates among KYB children. One of our major programs in the New York area begins to show a reduction in the onset of smoking (control schools 8% and study schools 4% after 5 years of intervention programs; Walter and Connolly 1985). Currently, our program begins in grade 1 and involves the entire school. We have not conducted such an effort for a sufficient length of time to measure its effect on cigarette smoking or tobacco chewing, though smoking-related attitude and knowledge have significantly improved early in the program.

While we are expanding the KYB concept across the United States and conducting pilot programs in Germany, Israel, and the People's Republic of China, it is our long-term strategy to have national or state legislatures provide appropriate legislation to make school health education programs mandatory. We must train teachers in health education, insist on health screening of all children, demand proper evaluation, and provide appropriate funding. Effective school health education, in respect to smoking, drugs, nutrition, dental hygiene, physical fitness, and teenage pregnan-

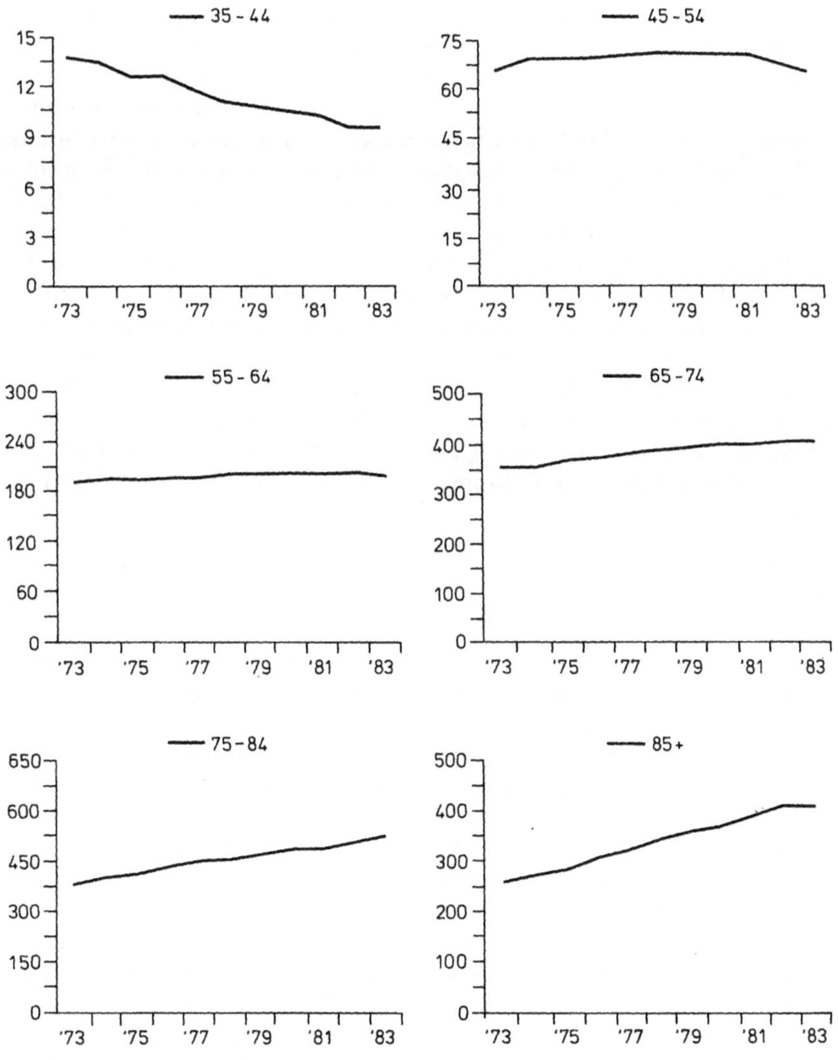

Fig. 6. Age-specific lung cancer mortality rates per 100000 white men. From Horm and Kessler (1986)

cy, is providing children with knowledge and self-esteem so that they can make the right health decisions. Thus, we can assist in giving our children the gift of health.

Changes in Lung Cancer Rates

The ultimate goal of preventive oncology is, of course, to reduce, if not eliminate the incidence of cancer. From that point of view, it is of some satisfaction to know that in younger men, though unfortunately less in younger women, the incidence as well as the mortality of lung cancer is decreasing. Most noticeably, this trend can be seen in Great Britain and now also in the United States. The decline of lung cancer, which is observed among men in the UK and in the USA is surely due in part to the fact that fewer young men are taking up the habit of cigarette smoking, and that more smokers among younger cohorts have quit than in previous decades (Fig. 6). The International Agency for Research on Cancer stated that the substantial decreases in lung cancer mortality which have recently been observed in middle-aged groups in the United Kingdom and Finland, have not been seen in other countries because the smoking habits which were initiated when these European cohorts were young adults became established long before the major reductions in smoke yields of cigarettes occurred (IARC 1986). However, this decline may also be due to a reduced tumor potential of low-yield cigarettes. It is likely that all three factors play a role with their relative effect for the overall reduction still to be determined. The future history of the lung cancer rate for women will help to evaluate the effect of low-yield cigarettes. The prevalence of smoking in younger age groups in women is at present stable. Their smoking rates will likely not reach the level of cigarette consumption by men two or three decades ago. Women smoke predominantly low-yield cigarettes. Thus, their rate of lung cancer will not be as high as that recorded for men. But death from lung cancer in women will continue to increase and is about to surpass the rate of deaths from breast cancer.

Epilogue

Man's triumphs against smallpox, typhus, and cholera were based on his ability to develop effective vaccines or sanitize the environment, measures relatively unaffected by the personal involvement of individuals. The prevention of tobacco-related diseases or, for that matter, cirrhosis of the liver and most cardiovascular events, require that all individuals change their lifestyles. For this new area of preventive lifestyle medicine to succeed, we need the full collaboration of the medical profession, the public, the schools and churches, work sites, media, industries that produce health-related products, government, and society as a whole.

We confront obstacles such as apathy of the public and the medical community, as well as vested commercial interests. The day must come when tobacco-related disease and notably, lung cancer will be as rare as they were at the beginning of the century. The true art of medicine does not lie in the ability to heal, but in the ability to prevent disease. As we examine opportunities in respect to tobacco-related diseases, we face a special and measurable challenge. On reflection, discovery appears easier than application, yet discovery is useless until and unless we act upon it.

References

Adler I (1912) Primary malignant growths of the lungs and bronchi. Longmans, Green, New York

American Cancer Society (1986) Cancer facts and figures. American Cancer Society, New York

American Health Foundation (1976) Symposium: the illusion of immortality – a dilemma of disease prevention. Prev Med 5:477–548

American Medical Association (1986) Statement by the House of Delegates. Annual meeting of the American Medical Association, 18 June, Chicago

Auerbach O, Hammond EC, Garfinkel L (1980) Changes in biomedical epithelium: then and now. Banbury Rep 3:141–154

Bernstein DF, Glasgow RE (1979) In: Pomerleau DF, Brady SP (eds) Behavioral medicine: theory and practice. Wilkins and Wilkins, pp 233–254

Borland BL, Rudolph JP (1975) Relative effects of low socio-economic status, parental smoking and poor scholastic performance on smoking among high school students. Soc Sci Med 9:27–30

DeVita V (1986) Annual report of the National Cancer Institute on the smoking, tobaco and cancer program. National Cancer Institute, US Department of Health and Human Services, NIH publication No 86-2687, April 1986

Dodds L, Davis S, Polissar L (1986) A population-based study of lung cancer incidence trends in histological type, 1974–81. JNCI 76:21–29

Doll R, Hill AB (1950) Smoking and carcinoma of the lung. Preliminary Report. Br Med J 2:739–748

Doll R, Peto R (1976) Mortality in relation to smoking: 20 years' observations on male British doctors. Br Med J 2(6051):1525–1536

Doll R, Peto R (1977) Mortality among doctors in different occupations. Br Med J 1(6074):1433–1436

Fagerström KO (1984) Effects of nicotine chewing gum and follow-up appointments in physician-based smoking cessation. Prev Med 13:517–527

Flay B (1985) Psychosocial approaches to smoking prevention: a review of findings. Health Psychol 4(5):449–488

Gritz ER, Baer-Weiss, Jarvik ME (1976) Titration of nicotine intake with full-length and half-length cigarettes. Clin Pharmacol Ther 20:552–556

Haley NJ, Sepkovic DW, Hoffmann D, Wynder EL (1985) Cigarette smoking as a risk for cardiovascular disease. Part V. Compensation with nicotine availability as a single variable. Clin Pharmacol Ther 38:164–170

Harris JE (1983) Cigarette smoking among successive birth cohorts of men and women in the United States during 1900–80. JNCI 71:473–479

Johnston LD, O'Malley PM, Bachman GG (1985) Use of licit and illicit drugs by America's high school students. National Institute on Drug Abuse. DHSS publication no (ADM) 85-1394, US Government Printing Office, Washington, DC

Hoffmann D, Hecht SS (1986) Perspectives in cancer research. Nicotine-derived N-nitrosamines and tobacco-related cancer: current status and future directions. Cancer Res 45:935–944

Horm JR, Kessler LG (1986) Falling rates of lung cancer in men in the United States. Lancet 1:425–426

IARC: International Agency for Research on Cancer (1986) Tobacco Smoking. IARC, Lyon, France (IARC Monographs on the evaluation of the carcinogenic risk of chemicals to humans, vol 38)

Levin ML, Goldstein H, Gerhardt PR (1950) Cancer and tobacco smoking. A preliminary report. JAMA 143:336–338

Melamed M, Flehinger B, Zaman MB et al. (1984) Screening for early lung cancer: results of the Memorial Sloan-Kettering Study in New York. Chest 86:44–53

Mohr U, Reznik G (1978) Tobacco carcinogenesis. In: Harris CC (ed) Pathogenesis and therapy of lung cancer. Dekker, New York, pp 263–367

Mueller FH (1939) Tabakmissbrauch und Lungencarcinom. Z Krebsforsch 49:57–84

National Center for Health Statistics (1985) Health United States 1984. US DHHS publication no (PHS) 85–1232, US Government Printing Office, Washington, DC

National Institute on Drug Abuse (1979) Cigarette smoking as a dependence process. In: Krasnegor NA (ed) NIDA research monograph 23. DHEW publication no (ADM) 79-800

Perry C, Killen J, Telch M, Slinkard LA, Danaher BG (1980) Peer-teaching smoking prevention among junior high students. Adolescence 9(58): 277–281

Royal College of Physicians (1962) Smoking and health. Summary of a report of the Royal College of Physicians of London on smoking in relation to cancer of the lung and other diseases. Pitman Medical, London

Russell MAH, Wilson C, Taylor C, Baker CD (1979) Effect of general practitioners' advice against smoking. Br Med J 2: 231–235

Schachter S (1978) Pharmacological and physiological determinant of smoking. Ann Intern Med 88: 104–114

Soemmering ST (1975) De mortis vasorum absorbentium corporis human. Varrentrapii et Wenneri, Traiectic and Moenum, Frankfurt/Main, Germany, p 109

US Department of Health, Education, and Welfare (1964) Smoking and health. Report of the advisory committee to the surgeon general of the public health service. USDHEW Public Health Service, publication no 1103

US Department of Health and Human Services (1981) Health consequences of smoking: the changing cigarette: a report of the surgeon general. US DHHS publication no 81-50154, US Government Printing Office, Washington, DC

US Department of Health and Human Services (1982) Student drug use in America 1975–1982. US DHHS publication no (ADM) 82-1221, US Government Printing Office, Washington, DC

US Department of Health and Human Services (1985) Use of licit and illicit drugs by America's high school students 1975–1984. US DHHS publication no (ADM) 85-1394, US Government Printing Office, Washington, DC

US Public Health Service, Office on Smoking and Health (1979) Smoking and health: a report of the surgeon general. US DHHS publication no (PHS) 79-50066, US Government Printing Office, Washington, DC

US Public Health Service (1984) the health consequences of smoking. A report of the surgeon general. DHHS publication no (PHS) 84-50205, pp 481–509, US Government Printing Office, Washington, DC

Vartianen E, Pallonen V, McAlister A, Koskela F, Puska P (1983) Effect of two years of education intervention in adolescent smoking. (The North Karelia youth project). Bull WHO 61(3): 529–532

Walter HJ, Connelly PA (1985) Screening for risk factors as a component of a chronic disease prevention program for youth. J School Health 55(5): 183–188

Walter HJ, Hofman A, Connelly PA, Barrett LT, Kost KL (1985) Primary prevention of chronic disease in childhood: changes in risk factors after one year of intervention. Am J Epidemiol 122(5): 772–781

Williams CL, Carter BJ, Arnold CB, Wynder EL (1979) Chronic disease risk factors among children: the "Know your body" study. J Chronic Dis 32: 505–513

Wohlford P (1970) Initiation of cigarette smoking: Is it related to parental smoking behavior? J Consult Clin Psychol 34: 148–151

Wynder EL, Graham EA (1950) Tobacco smoking as a possible etiological factor in bronchiogenic carcinoma. A study of six hundred and eighty-four proven cases. J Am Med Assoc 143: 329–336

Wynder EL, Hoffmann D (1967) Tobacco and tobacco smoke. Studies in experimental carcinogenesis. Academic, New York

Summary of Discussion: Session 3

H.-G. Neumann

It is possible to apply legal, technical, and personal measures to eliminate risk factors before they cause an effect. As a legal measure the control of food additives has been mentioned, but the role of food as such and the preventive effects of low fat and high-fiber diets as a personal measure were not covered. Although some feel that macronutrients play an important role as tumor enhancers, others see some circumstantial evidence but no proof of such a correlation.

In China some high risk areas for certain types of tumors have been identified. The high incidence of esophageal carcinoma for instance has been attributed to nitrosamine exposure and a dietary deficiency in vitamin A. A 5-year intervention study, in which vitamin A was supplemented in the diet of part of the population, did not show any effect on tumor incidence. Up to now intervention studies of this type in China have produced negative results. It was also discussed whether antioxidants should be added to food on a larger scale in order to inactivate metabolically formed radicals and reactive oxygen species. But some of the antioxidants are suspected to be tumor promoters in their own right and more information is necessary about the dose dependence of the desired and undesired effects before this idea should be considered any further. Furthermore, the intentional supplementation of food for this purpose would be against the law in this country.

Extending the discussion about the prevention of occupational health hazards, it was stressed that in addition to cancer, chronic lung disease and neurological disorders deserve some attention, and the relative importance of these chronic health problems should be assessed.

With regard to assessing the possible carcinogenic risk of chemicals it was noted that relevant information is lacking in many cases. Although test results are now required by law before the introduction of bulk chemicals in Europe, patent laws were said to prevent early publication of all the available information. However, there remains a need for more data on which the assessment of the carcinogenic potential can be based both for bulk chemicals as well as for minor products, and a distinction between these two categories should actually not be made.

Primary prevention carried out by substituting a proven carcinogen by a less well-characterized product may only produce new problems. Glass fibers as a substitute for asbestos are a case in point. It was quoted that a recent discussion at the IARC did not lead to a decision. There are positive test results with glass fibers and epidemiological studies of other possible substitutes have not even been started.

A final suggestion of how to improve occupational health protection underlined the necessity of combining epidemiology with biomonitoring procedures particularly to identify new risk groups. All workers at risk should be registered and the individual exposures to the chemicals in question measured.

Although there appears to exist a general agreement that cigarette smoking is the predominant cause for lung cancer and primary prevention is best achieved by stopping this hazardous habit, there are different opinions on many of the details. A difficulty in the development of a less hazardous cigarette is the fact that nicotine itself can be nitrosated and thus activated to powerful carcinogens, which could contribute significantly to the overall genotoxic exposure. This is not reduced by lowering the tar fraction, but may possibly be influenced by the content of nitrate which could also be lowered.

Smokers generally develop Kreyberg I-type lung tumors. Presently, a decrease of these tumors and an increase of Kreyberg II-type lung tumors is being noted. Although this could be explained by changes in smoking habits, it has also been emphasized that this may point to a role of other causes for the development of lung cancer.

SESSION 4

Physical Carcinogens

Chairman: W. GÖSSNER

Cancer Risk from Ultraviolet Radiation

H. Ippen

All the world cares about the prevention of cruelty to animals, about saving them from the clutches of the vivisectionists, yet no one seems concerned about hundreds of thousands of mishandled children and battered babies. The case is similar with respect to cancer risks. The largely improbable cancer risk due to traces of formaldehyde in our environment is publicized extensively by the mass media while the certain genesis of skin cancer by light (Blum 1959; Urbach et al. 1974; Urbach 1982; Vitaliano et al. 1980) gets virtually no public attention. The best prevention of this highest of all cancer risks can, therefore, only be achieved in the untiring and patient education of the public by scientists and medical men.

Today the risk of cancer through exposure to ultraviolet light can be viewed as established. Statistics and clinical findings speak a common language. The most frequent malignant tumor of the skin, the basal cell carcinoma, is to be found predominantly in the chronically exposed and light-damaged facial region. Its precursors are the light-induced degeneration of subcutaneous connective tissue (basophilic degeneration and elastosis) and possibly also solar keratoses. The more seldom encountered squamous cell carcinoma of the skin may also develop in chronically light-exposed regions, whereby actinic keratoses and cornua cutanea may be initial stages of such malignant development. In contrast, cancer of the lower lip is far more often found, normally preceded by the actinic cheilitis. In this context an involuntary mass experiment deserves mention. At the beginning of this century lip cancer in Turkey was found exclusively among men since women were forbidden to go outdoors unveiled. Legal prohibition of the veil by Kemal Ataturk led to lip cancer among women within a few years.

Another type of tumor that develops predominantly in light-damaged skin is the lentigo maligna which can give rise to the malignant melanoma. The superficial spreading melanoma presently seems to be on the increase. It shows such dramatic differences of distribution between men and women that the influence of light must necessarily be discussed. The superficial spreading melanoma in men is primarily found on the upper torso, whilst in women it occurs largely on the lower legs, where sometimes it even develops multiply. While some authors (Braun-Falco and Landthaler 1986; Elwood et al. 1985; Fitzpatrick and Sober 1985; Green et al. 1985; Illig et al. 1986; Korting 1986; Lew et al. 1983) discussed these findings in connection with severe sunburns of these areas, in my opinion, it is necessary to regard the summation of numerous slight actinic damage to the males' largely unclothed upper body and the females' (at least those not of the pants-suit generations) legs and calves. Finally, the keratoacanthoma, also occurring in chronically light-exposed skin, not infrequently progressing to squamous cell carcinoma, must also be mentioned.

On the basis of clinical and epidemiological observations concerning the relationship of cancer frequency and geographic latitude, and, as is the case with Australia observation of a rather homogeneous population, a clear-cut causal relationship between light exposure and skin cancer has been established. Nonetheless, a certain hereditary factor, of equal importance, should be contrasted with individual light sensitivity of the skin in conjunction with the degree of solar exposure. Clinical observations and epidemiological studies have shown a decrease in the risk of skin cancer with increasing pigment content of the skin. An example of the foregoing is the fact that the Celtic type, with both little and poor pheomelanin and a thin horny layer, develops light-induced cancer far more often than the Mediterranean type, or even the black African, both of whom have a higher skin content of eumelanin and a thicker horny layer. A nomogram can be developed using these determinants, i.e., degree of light exposure and constitutional light sensitivity of the skin in order to determine the light-induced cancer risk. This nomogram shows the photosensitive Australian immigrant in an equatorial climate to have the highest and the Negro at the polar cap the lowest risk of developing cancer.

Despite the fact that I have spoken only of light as a carcinogenic factor, I tried to suggest by my title the carcinogenic effect of a small spectral band of sunlight. This undoubtedly means ultraviolet, the short wave part of the spectrum. Probably the shorter the wave length, the greater the carcinogenic potential of ultraviolet light due to its increasing quantum energy. Hereby the degree of penetration of the skin, and more particularly of the horny layer, should be considered. With the decrease in wave length, this penetration also rashly decreases so that long-wave ultraviolet A has a relatively high proportion, ultraviolet B much less, and ultraviolet C only a small amount of energy which reaches living cells. The other limiting factor is, of course, the spectral composition of terrestrial sunlight, which has its short wave extreme at about 295 nm. The maximum carcinogenic effect of sunlight seems to lie at about 300 nm, while the theoretical maximum of artificial light sources would be at about 280 nm. A new upper limit of the carcinogenic ultraviolet effect may be provisionally established at about 335 nm.

In my opinion, as a consequence of the limits of our measurement instruments a simple calculation is left out of consideration. If one assumes that within a particular time 10^{15} ultraviolet quanta strike the skin, and if we are able to establish with a very sensitive detection device that the portion of UV B is less than 0.1%, then more than 10^{10} UV B quanta reach the surface of the skin. In view of the assumed penetration of 1% at least 10^{8} UV B quanta reach living cells. This consideration seems to me not only important in respect to the reputedly UV B-free artificial light sources, but also meaningful in regard to investigations concerning the effects of ultraviolet A in the skin. Berger was able to demonstrate in nude mice that pure UV A produces dramatic connective tissue damage as light-induced elastosis. On the other hand, if his light source emitted even demonstrable UV B, then the experimental animals regularly developed malignant tumors. In this context the question of photo-augmentation, of an enhancement effect of small UV B amounts by large UV A exposure, arises. It can be assumed that UV B is the carcinogen, but that the more predominant solar UV A, which penetrates deeper into the skin, is probably a cofactor. It could be discussed as to whether the skin is prepared for malignant differentiation by the UV A-induced connective tissue damage, as well as the synergistic effects of both types of radiation, in the sense of enhancement of the carcinogenic effect of UV B quanta by simultaneously penetrating UV A quanta.

We may assume from necessary considerations concerning prevention of particularly important environmental carcinogens that regular exposure of susceptible individuals to UV B (and possibly also UV A) must necessarily lead to the occurrence of malignant tumors in the predominantly light-exposed skin areas, i.e., face, neck, and backs of the hands. With increasing light exposure, this risk increases dramatically according to individual light sensitivity. Prevention seems to be relatively simple. Those endangered individuals should avoid unnecessary light exposure, particularly of those skin regions which unavoidably get large UV B doses in the course of life. This is possible with the right kind of clothing, i.e., gloves, floppy hats, and sun umbrellas. Additionally a large selection of effective sunscreens is available. But in a majority of the Europeans unconscious and emotional factors seem to be stronger than intellectual application of facts which are after all well known. The situation is comparable to that of physicians, who despite their knowledge of the connections between lung cancer and cigarettes, do not give up smoking.

When closely questioned, most people will admit that sunlight causes skin damage. Some of them even realize that it is carcinogenic. But when pressed the latter either proclaim that only an excess is dangerous, or mystical associations and psychosocial fabrications are offered in explanation. These mystical associations are maintained by the life-giving blessings of sunlight which are part of the objectively and subjectively advantageous effects. But unfortunately even intelligent people often arrive at the conclusion that something so beneficial can hardly be deleterious. Even more dangerous than such mystification and concomitant repression of solar-induced carcinogenic risk are psychic factors and social compunctions, which seem to exist for the pale-faced civilized man.

The positive feelings connected with sunbathing give expression to the compulsive desire for tanned skin as a visible expression of health, youth, sportiveness, and the material prerequisites for travel to sunny climates. Naturally, but paradoxically, the desire for well-tanned skin seems most predominant amongst those people who have the least capability for tanning (Fitzpatrick's skin types I and II, in whom even a short sunbath can induce massive acute skin damage in the sense of blistering sunburn). These are the people most highly threatened by skin cancer. The whole problem of light-induced skin cancer, as the most frequently induced exogeneous malignant tumor, could be easily solved if one were to succeed in freeing the "Caucasian" from the psychosocial compunction to have a deep brown tan. We are far from this goal as is proven by the boom that artificial light sources have had as "skin tanners" in our countries in the past few years. Whether and to what extent such solariums are responsible for the occurrence of malignant skin tumors can first be decided in the years to come since the latent, or dormant, period until occurrence of basal cell and squamous cell cancers, even in highly skin sensitive and heavily light-exposed persons, is unfortunately very long.

The wish to have a well-tanned skin, which in contrast to nineteenth century preferences first became desirable in our time, has often been criticized by intelligent people. Yet the beneficial effect of light on the human body, its metabolism and the psyche are offered as excuses for indulging this wish by the very same people. As soon as one suggests sunning the whole body with the exception of the endangered regions, i.e., face, neck, hands, and lower arms, which then should receive a textile protection or sunblockers, the real reason becomes apparent, compulsion to tanning of the continuously exposed and readily shown skin regions.

It may be deduced that our present-day knowledge does allow a substantial reduction of tumor risk through natural and artificial light sources. To accomplish this, intensive education of the public would necessarily have to include the following aspects:

1. At highest risk, apart from those people with pathological conditions such as xeroderma pigmentosum (a repair-system defect) and albinism (absence of melanin synthesis), are people whose skin contains little or no pigment, which when present is of the phaeomelanin type. This is clearly the case in the so-called Celtic types. These individuals are not only the strawberry blonds, but may even have brown eyes and dark hair, always displaying a reddish tinge in direct sunlight. Northern European blue-eyed blonds are appearently less endangered due to the predominance of eumelanin. At the other end of the danger scale are blacks who develop light-induced malignant tumors only in their albinos.
2. The second most important risk factor after individual (racial) light sensitivity is the summation of ultraviolet light collected during the course of life. This total amount consists of two components.

   a) The often highly divergent degrees of lifelong exposure to light of certain skin regions may be characterized as largest for portions of the head and smallest for the insides of the upper arms, armpits, insides of the thighs, and the skinfold between the buttocks. When regarding the head and neck, pronounced differences are due in part to anatomy and in part to fashion. The nose, cheek bones, and forehead are substantially more exposed than the chin shadows. Androgenetic alopecia brings along a particularly large risk since hair loss involves continuous solar exposure of the bald head at every angle of the sun, because sunlight then always falls perpendicularly on some part of the head. And as long as men wear shorter hair than women, the male nape of the neck will exhibit more substantial skin changes. Correspondingly women then exhibit these changes at the v-necked exposure of the bust. Similar findings in women existed for the lower legs, at least as long as skirts and nylon stockings were fashionable. The clothing habits of the blue-jeans' generation have already begun to mask this difference. Hands and lower arms are practically only endangered at the extensor aspects. The thick horny layer of the palms of the hands effectively protccts against both chronic and acute light-induced skin damage. Finally, it should be mentioned that certain endangered skin regions are those of particular occupations or sport affecionados, i.e., swim coaches, life-guards, and athletes. These persons often develop malignant skin tumors of the upper torso and lateral aspects of the thighs.

   b) Besides the varying light exposure of different skin regions during the course of life, the intensity of sunbathing will affect the outcome. This intensity depends primarily on the elevation of the sun, type of cloud cover, and the immediate surroundings, i.e., water, sand, and snow. The height of the sun depends upon the degree of latitude, the time of day, and the season of the year. The sun elevation in all latitudes is highest at twelve o'clock. The sun is most dangerous between the hours of 10:00 a.m. and 2:00 p.m., local time. The further one travels from the equator, the larger the effect of the season of the year. This means that in our latitude the longest day of the year ± 6 weeks, i.e., from the beginning of May until the end of July, is the most dangerous time. One must also consider the phenomenon of light habituation, that continuous decrease in light sensitivity through increased thickness of the horny layer (Miescher's "light-induced callus"). This means that the same amount of light is more dangerous in the spring than in the fall.

The haziness of the sky is often incorrectly estimated. With a slightly clouded sky the relationship between direct solar and indirect, "heavenly," or reflected radiation of the murky atmosphere can be so skewed that one gets a sunburn in the shade nearly as quickly as in the sun. Water droplets in the sky can increase reflection of the sunlight substantially. The same is also true for the immediate surroundings, such as snow, foamy waters, white beach sand, or even fog.

If one were to consider all of the foregoing, then the most substantial reduction of the risk of UV-induced cancer for the Caucasian could be accomplished through the following:

1. Avoidance of any unnecessary exposure to the sun of the regularly exposed skin regions of the head, neck, and lower arms through the use of protective clothing and sunblockers. The so-called broad-spectrum sunscreens should include substantial amounts of UV A filters. This point is of particular importance for all those engaged in outdoor occupations, e.g., farmworkers, seamen, construction workers, and roadmen.
2. Leisure time activities and sporting events should be held in the early morning or late afternoon and not during the midday heat.
3. To partake of the undoubtedly numerous beneficial effects of sunlight, that 90% of the surface area of the skin should be utilized which is not regularly exposed. But even here there must be limits.
4. The present desire and compulsion for tanning should be viewed as a problem and solved. Intensive effort and research for the development of really satisfactory artificial skin tanners is necessary. With these skin-tanning agents, a chemical reaction in the horny layer leads to the brown color, thus circumventing the risky new production and darkening of the skin pigment, melanin.

I am afraid, however, that these considerations will remain unfulfilled wishes. We will probably have to live with a known and proven cancer risk which will continue to be on the increase through more travel fever, more free time, more artificial light, and even continuous repression of reasonable considerations.

References

Blum HF (1959) Carcinogenesis by ultraviolet light. Princeton University Press, Princeton

Braun-Falco O, Landthaler M (1986) Gibt es eine gesicherte kausalpathogenetische Verbindung von Sonnenlicht und Melanom? Med Welt 37:815–816

Elwood JM et al (1985) Cutaneous melanoma in relation to intermittent and constant sun exposure. The Western Canada melanoma study. Int J Cancer 35:427–433

Fitzpatrick TB, Sober AJ (1985) Sunlight and skin cancer. N Engl J Med 313:818–819
Green A et al. (1985) Sunburn and malignant melanoma. Br J Cancer 51:393–397
Illig L (1986) Gibt es eine gesicherte kausalpathogenetische Verbindung von Sonnenlicht und Melanom? Med Welt 37:816–817
Korting GW (1986) Gibt es eine gesicherte kausalpathogenetische Verbindung von Sonnenlicht und Melanom? Med Welt 37:817
Lew RA et al (1983) Sun exposure habits in patients with cutaneous melanoma: a case control study. J Dermatol Surg Oncol 9:981–986
Urbach F (1982) Epidemiology and etiology of skin cancer in man. In: Grundmann E (ed) Cancer epidemiology. Fischer, Stuttgart (Cancer campaign, vol 6)
Urbach F et al (1974) Ultraviolet carcinogenesis: experimental, global, and genetic aspects. In: Pathak MA et al (eds) Sunlight and man. University of Tokyo Press, Tokyo
Vitaliano PP et al (1980) The relative importance of risk factors in nonmelanoma carcinoma. Arch Dermatol 116:454–456

Assessment of Cancer Risks Due to Ionizing Radiations

A. M. Kellerer

Introduction

The enduring controversy on nuclear energy and the recent reactor accident have made ionizing radiation one of the most widely discussed tumor-inducing agents, although compared with major contributors, such as tobacco, its role appears to be minor. There is also little doubt that ionizing radiation is probably the one carcinogen which has been most extensively studied. X-rays were discovered in 1895, and 17 years passed before physicists began to understand their nature. But it took merely a few weeks before the first skin lesions were seen, and only 7 years before an X-ray induced skin cancer was recognized (Frieben 1902). In 1911 when Max von Laue obtained the first X-ray diffraction patterns in Munich, von Jagie et al. (1911) in Berlin reported a cluster of five leukemias in radiologists. The lesson was learned slowly. The hands of radiologists were less widely used as routine test objects for focusing the X-ray equipment, but scattered radiation or even the primary beam were not generally avoided, and before long leukemia became the professional affliction of radiologists.

A first dose limit was set in 1921 in terms of an observable skin reaction, a level 100 times the present limits. In 1928 the International Commission for Radiological Protection (ICRP) was founded, just 1 year after H. J. Muller (1927) had shown the mutagenic potential of X-rays and the apparent absence of a threshold. At the time the limit for radiation workers was set at 6 roentgen per month, a dose roughly comparable to 0.06 Sv per month, in today's units. The value was about 15 times higher than present limits, and adherence to the regulations may then have been far below present standards. The prevailing philosophy was still, that tumors could be induced by radiation only after a persistent accumulation of high radiation doses.

As a little-known aside of some historical interest one may note that Giachino Failla, the distinguished radiologist and physicist, had recommended at the time a "tolerance dose rate" of 0.6 roentgen per month, a value nearly equal to today's limit. The proposal was based on animal and human data (Failla 1932). He "had at the hospital a canary which has been continuously (day and night) in a beam of X-rays for about five months... In this time the bird has received about 6000 roentgen of hard X-rays without apparent deleterious effects." However, Failla was also aware of effects that may develop later, hence the need for an epidemiological study – also of modest proportions. Three of his technicians were in charge of administering the 4 g radium pack at Memorial Hospital. Averaging over several years a dose of roughly 0.6 roentgen per month, they exhibited no substantial depression of white blood counts and no degree of lowered vitality. Thus, the limit seemed appropriate.

Between 1920 and 1930, and even later, appalling misuses of X-rays – even their utilization to terminate pregnancies – were still common. Treatment of benign conditions with X-rays or radionuclides was fairly general, which led to a wide range of observations on radiation-induced tumors (UNSCEAR 1977; NAS/NRC 1980). Diagnostic application of X-rays and technical uses of radionuclides were other areas where little or no concern was given to radiation protection.

Former Misuses of Radionuclides

The tragic heritage of the misuses of ionizing radiation in three main fields of application can be seen in the fate of patients treated with the short-lived radium-224, of patients (mostly soldiers) subjected to angiography with the α-emitting contrast medium thorotrast, and in industrial workers (mostly young women) who incorporated large amounts of radium-226 and radium-228 when they painted luminous dials. A brief consideration of these experiences may help to put some of the present problems and anxieties into perspective.

The last-named example concerns the most disastrous industrial misuse of a radionuclide. There were nearly 2000 workers, in the United States alone, who painted luminous watch dials with the long-lived radium-226. These workers, mostly young girls, were paid by the piece, and consequently they used the quickest method to sharpen the tips of the brushes. Employing their lips to sharpen the brushes they ingested large amounts of the radium paint. The high doses of incorporated radium led to numerous osteosarcomas and carcinomas of the paranasal sinuses or mastoids. Up to 1983, these tumors had contributed 12% of all deaths that have occurred in those whose radium intake has been measured. The Center of Human Radiobiology at Argonne National Laboratory has been in charge of the epidemiological study (Rundo et al. 1986); it has recently been reduced to a size which will make it nearly impossible to continue a valid follow-up of the fate of the dial painters. The resulting loss of singular medical and scientific information will be irreversible as well as indefensible.

The dentist of one of the dial painters first assumed red phosphorus to be a component of the luminous paint and blamed it for his patient's grave jaw damage. When this explanation failed, he continued to search for an explanation. Harrison Martland, whom he had consulted, focused his suspicion on radium-226. When this became known, he received an angry letter from Mme Curie; herself a victim of radiation, she called him a charlatan for failing to acknowledge that radiation can do no harm except at very large doses (Merril Eisenbud, personal communication). Although the letter has been lost, it remains a telling sign of the lack of appreciation of radiation risks in the first half of this century.

Decades later an equally tragic misuse of an α-emitting radionuclide occurred in Germany where, at a private clinic shortly after the Second World War, numerous children with bone tuberculosis were injected with large amounts of radium-224 and where the same treatment was given to adults with ankylosing spondylitis (Morbus Bechterew). The fate of the patients might never have become known, except for the actions of a young pediatrician who observed the treatment and spoke out against it. Heinz Spiess secured against the opposition of the director of the clinic the patient data and he has, jointly with Charles Mays, conducted one of the most important studies of a group of patients subjected to the effects of ionizing radiations (Mays et al. 1986). Unlike the British ankylosing spondylitis patients who were treated with X-rays and developed, as Court Brown and Doll (1956) and Smith and Doll (1982) have demonstrated, an excess rate of leukemias and other tumors, the radium-224 patients incurred a large number of osteosarcomas. There were more than 50 osteosarcomas in the group of roughly 800 patients who were followed. Among the children with the largest doses, the rate of osteosarcomas was extremely high. Radium-224 has a short half-time of only 3.5 days, and the temporal pattern of the occurrence of osteosarcomas is, therefore, the undistorted response to irradiations fractionated over treatment periods of only several months. A maximum of the rate of osteosarcomas was found 5 to 10 years after the treatment, in later years the number of cases has declined. The quantitative analysis of the data has led to a linear-quadratic dose dependence with the risk estimate of $8.5 \cdot 10^{-3}$ per gray of mean skeletal dose (Chmelevsky et al. 1986). The study has been extended now to include various other types of radiation damage, including radiation-induced cataracts.

The observations on the radium-224 patients are directly relevant to a continuing medical practice. Treatment of ankylosing spondylitis with radium-224 is still practised in Germany, but far lower doses are given which amount to a mean skeletal dose of less than 1 gray. The osteosarcoma risk from this treatment would appear to be less than 1% according to the results of the Spiess study. The continued epidemiological investigation of the low dose treatment is consistent with this estimate (Wick et al. 1986). Despite the remaining hazard of osteosarcoma induction, there are valid arguments to defend the present-day radium-224 treatment of ankylosing spondylitis.

The deplorable consequences of another major misuse of a radionuclide are being studied in Heidelberg by von Kaick and his colleagues (1986). Thorotrast was probably the best contrast medium ever available for angiography. However, it contained thorium-232, an α-emitter of extremely long life time. Although numerous lives were saved by the use of thorotrast, it is by now inconceivable that thorotrast was still utilized up to and even beyond 1950. A number of scientists in different countries have studied, and are still studying, the effects of thorotrast which stays in the tissue and blood vessels of the patients, and which has caused a large number of liver tumors. For the remaining patients, liver tumors are now responsible for roughly half of all deaths.

Observation of the Atomic Bomb Survivors and the Estimation of Risk Coefficients

The main source of knowledge on radiation-induced tumors has been and continues to be the fate of the survivors of the atomic bombings. Studies have been performed during the past 40 years, first by the Atomic Bomb Casuality Commission (ABCC) and later by the Radiation Effects Research Foundation (RERF) in Hiroshima (see Yoshimoto et al. 1981; Ellett et al. 1985). The Life Span Study sample (LSS) contains about 60000 survivors of the bombing in Hiroshima and about 30000 survivors of the bombing in Nagasaki. When the bombs were used against Japan no radiation effects were foreseen, since those who would be highly exposed were expected not to survive the heat and the blast.

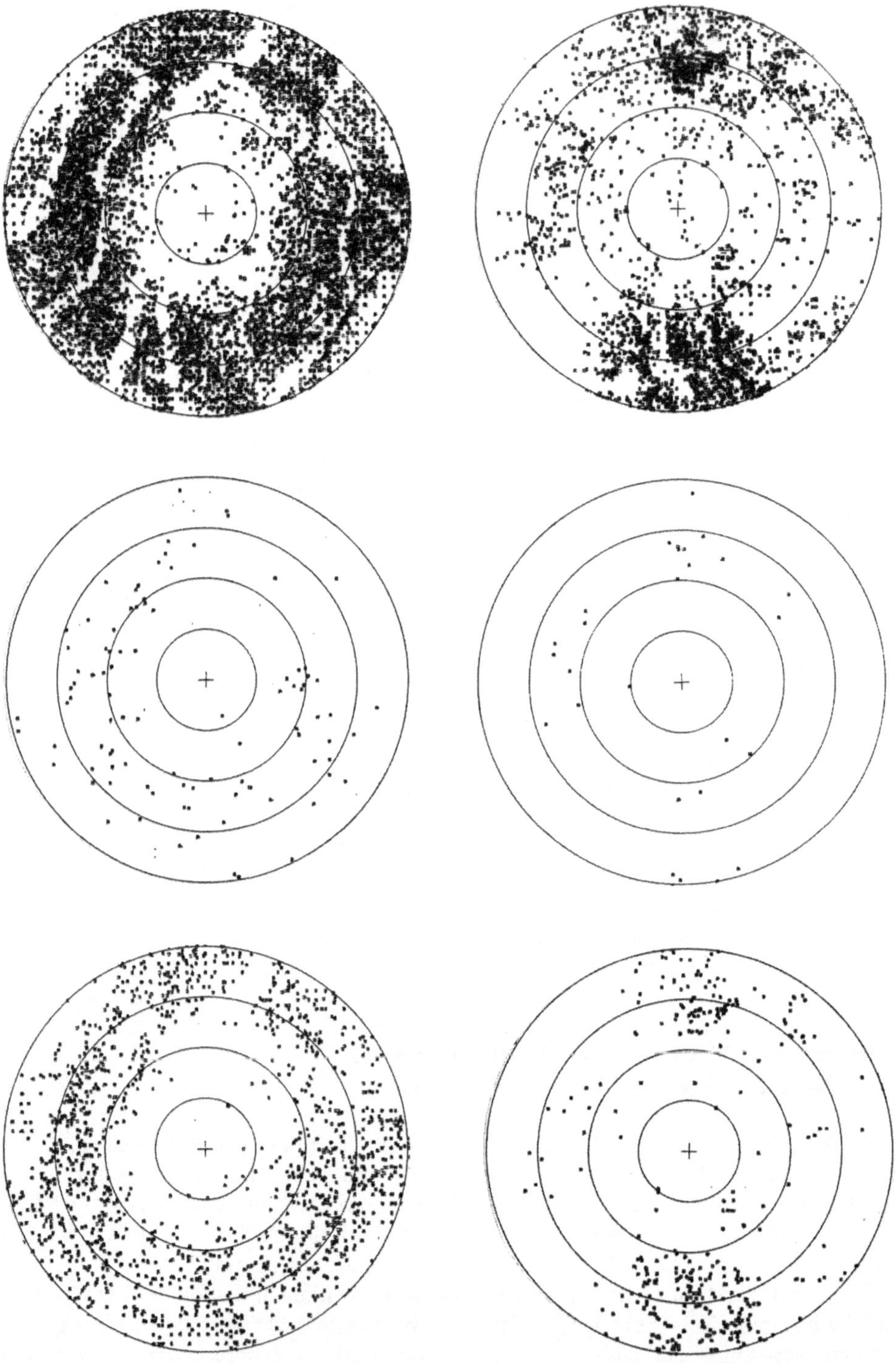

The diagrams of Fig. 1 show the positions of the survivors at the time of the bombing up to a distance of 2000 m from the hypocenters; they also show the extent of acute deaths at smaller distances and the number of cancer and leukemia deaths. Against expectation, and after merely a few years, leukemias appeared in excessive numbers among the survivors in Hiroshima and Nagasaki. The excess rates were so high that almost all leukemias among the highly exposed and about half of all leukemias recorded in the diagrams are due to the irradiation. These observations, the earlier data on the British ankylosing spondylitis patients (Court Brown and Doll 1956), and the leukemias in radiologists led E. B. Lewis to the hypothesis that leukemia could result from a radiation-induced mutation in a single blood-forming cell and to the assumption that the incidence of cancers might increase as a linear function of dose without threshold (Lewis 1957, 1963). At the time, this assumption was less controversial than it is nowadays, because it was still held that hereditary damage was the principle hazard of low doses of ionizing radiations.

Subsequent studies, mainly on the survivors of the atomic bombings and among the British ankylosing spondylitis patients, have provided a wide range of data on various tumors produced by ionizing radiations in man. For solid tumors, the relative increase of the spontanous rates turned out to be much lower than for leukemia. But the total number of cases is sufficiently large to derive dose dependences for tumors of various organs. Although significant excesses have been seen only at doses of about 1 Gy or more, risk coefficients have been derived which are now applied to very small doses. Table 1 contains risk coefficients presented by ICRP (1977), and a few essential observations must be made.

First, the numerical values of the risk coefficients are such that the total risk for life-time cancer mortality exceeds the risk for hereditary damage. In fact, the comparison can only be valid if a dose dependence without threshold is assumed for radiation-induced tumors. The ICRP has made this assumption, and has made it the basis of its radiation protection philosophy.

In the present context it is interesting to note that hereditary damage due to ionizing radiation has never been demonstrated in man, not even in the descendants of the survivors from Hiroshima and Nagasaki. Great efforts have been made and are still being made to demonstrate the genetic effects. Plans are considered, at present, to supplement past work on protein analysis by an extensive program of DNA studies. That past efforts have failed to demonstrate genetic effects of the irradiation is due to the predominance of other factors which mask the small expected increments. It is, nevertheless, agreed that hereditary effects are caused by ionizing radiations and that they are produced without a threshold of dose. One can, furthermore, assume that the numerical estimates of the risk coefficients are of the right order of magnitude.

For radiation carcinogenesis the situation is reversed. There is a wealth of data, but the extrapolation to low doses remains a conjecture. The linear hypothesis can

---

Fig. 1. Coordinate plots (Yoshimoto et al. 1981) of the persons in the LSS sample who were within 2000 m of the hypocenters at the bombing of Hiroshima *(left column)* and Nagasaki *(right column)*. *Upper row,* all persons in LSS sample; *intermediate row,* all leukemia deaths till 1978, *bottom row,* all cancer deaths (except leukemia) till 1978.

Preliminary estimates (Ellett et al. 1985) of kerma in free air distances 1000 m, 1500 m, 2000 m: Hiroshima, 5.3 Gy, 0.65 Gy, 0.07 Gy; Nagasaki, 10 Gy, 1.2 Gy, 0.16 Gy

Table 1. Risk coefficients of ICRP (averaged over age and sex)

Life-time mortality of cancer	Per Sievert
Leukemia	0.002
Mammary tumors	0.0025
Lung cancer	0.002
Osteosarcoma	0.0005
Thyroid tumors	0.0005
Other organs	0.005
	0.0125
Severe hereditary damage (2 generations)	0.004

neither be proved nor disproved at present, and it remains uncertain whether improved knowledge of the molecular mechanisms of cellular transformations will ever settle the question.

Basic principles of microdosimetry permit the statement that radiation effects on individual cells can have no threshold in dose and that their probability must be proportional to dose at low doses (Kellerer and Rossi 1982). This is so because energy is transferred to the cells by individual charged particles. At sufficiently low doses – fractions of one milligray for sparsely ionizing radiations and several milligray for densely ionizing radiations – only few cells are traversed by a charged particle. The dose determines then merely the number of cells affected, but not the energy deposition to these cells. Effects on autonomous cells must therefore be proportional to the number of cells affected and thus to dose. The statement remains valid even if the possible, and still largely unknown, role of various intracellular DNA-repair systems is taken into account. Somatic mutations are, therefore, produced without a threshold of dose. However, host factors, i.e., effects on the tissue level, may depend on dose in a way which can not be predicted. Their possible contribution to the progression of a transformed cell towards the growth of a tumor remains unknown.

A second statement on risk factors must be added. Although the estimates are largely based on the observation of the survivors of the atomic bombings, they are consistent with a wide range of studies from the medical application of X-rays. If the atomic bombings had not taken place, there would still be risk estimates of the same order of magnitude. It is less certain whether there would be the ICRP philosophy of linearity for radiation-induced tumors. However, this is the prevailing philosophy in radiation protection, and it has important implications.

Definition of the Effective Dose

For the consideration of risk factors, a few technical notions are required. The first concept is that of dose equivalent which equals absorbed dose of radiation multiplied

Table 2. Weight factors[a] representing the contribution of each organ to the risk of hereditary damage or mortality from radiation-induced tumors

i		w_i
1	Gonads	0.25
2	Breast	0.15
3	Red bone marrow	0.12
4	Lung	0.12
5	Thyroid	0.03
6	Bone surfaces	0.03
7	Remaining organs	0.30

[a] They equal the risk coefficients (see Table 1) normalized to their sum

Definition of effective dose:

$$H_{\mathrm{eff}} = \sum_{i=1}^{7} w_i H_i$$

where H_i is the mean dose equivalent to the organ i, and w_i is the weight factor for this organ

by a quality factor. The quality factor is, by convention, defined as a function of the linear energy transfer of charged particles and it accounts for the assumed biological effectiveness of a radiation at small doses. It is set equal to unity for all sparsely ionizing radiations, i.e., for γ-rays, X-rays, or electrons. Roughly speaking, it is equal to 10 for neutrons which transfer energy to the exposed material by releasing densely ionizing recoil nuclei. It is approximately 20 for α-particles which are also densely ionizing and produce thousands of ionizations while they traverse a cell nucleus. To avoid confusion, one has chosen the special name gray (Gy) for the unit J/kg when it is used with absorbed dose, while the special name sievert (Sv) is used when the unit is applied to dose equivalent.[1] There are proposals, at present, to change the values of the quality factor (ICRU 1986). This is likely to be a controversial topic in radiation protection in the years to come, and it is a question closely linked to the remaining uncertainties of risk assessment and to the lack of human data for the effects of neutrons.

When the body is exposed uniformly, the meaning of the dose or the dose equivalent is clear. When the body is exposed nonuniformly, or when certain organs only are exposed, more complicated specifications of dose are required. To provide a single quantity which can adequately express the resulting overall level of exposure, one has introduced the effective dose equivalent (ICRP 1977), which is now usually called the effective dose. It is a weighted average of all the organ doses. The weighting factor for each organ represents its fractional contribution to the total somatic and genetic risk (see Table 2). The notion may appear artificial, but it is, in fact, a

[1] The former units rad (1 rad = 0.01 Gy) and rem (1 rem = 0.01 Sv) are still widely used

natural matter, if one assumes proportionality to dose at low doses for radiation-induced tumors.

For clarification and illustration one may use an example familiar from the discussion after the reactor accident. The weighting factor for the thyroid is 0.03. If a child consumes a liter of milk contaminated with 1000 Bq of iodine-131, about half of the activity may be collected in the thyroid and it produces there a dose equivalent of roughly 3 mSv. Multiplication by the weighting factor results in an effective dose of roughly 0.1 mSv. For the purposes of radiation protection it is assumed that the exposure of the thyroid to 3 mSv causes a risk of the same magnitude as a whole body exposure of 0.1 mSv which may be caused, for example, by external γ-irradiation or by incorporation of cesium-137.

Validity of the Risk Estimates and Applicability of the Assessment System

One can ask two questions. First, how reliable are the risk coefficients? Second, how useful are they? An adequate answer to either question is outside the scope of the present survey. However, a brief summary can be given.

There has been occasion, in recent years, to doubt the validity of the risk estimates. The reason is that the dosimetry for the atomic bomb explosions has turned out to be incorrect (Loewe and Mendelsohn 1981). Some years ago it was thought that the larger part of the radiation effects in Hiroshima were due to neutrons emitted by the uranium bomb (Rossi and Kellerer 1974; Rossi and Mays 1978). In Nagasaki there were hardly any neutrons, because the plutonium bomb was surrounded by tons of conventional explosives, which shielded the emitted neutrons effectively. The revision of the dosimetry, while not finally concluded, has now led to the consensus that even in Hiroshima there were few neutrons. It was argued then, that effects earlier ascribed to neutrons must now be assigned to γ-rays, with a resulting increase of the risk estimates. However, the revised dosimetry has led to increased γ-doses in Hiroshima (Ellett et al. 1985), and this balances largely the disappearance of neutrons. Any resulting change of the risk estimates due to the revision of the Japanese dosimetry would appear to be less than a factor of 2.

A more substantial change of the risk estimates may arise if the excess rates of mammary tumors, thyroid tumors, lung tumors, and of intestinal tumors persist, and if they follow the increases of the spontaneous rates in the aging collective of exposed persons. The term relative risk model refers to such a persistence and age-dependent increase of excess tumor rates. The Japanese data appear to be in line with a relative risk model, and this appearance is underscored by the occurrence of breast cancer in recent years in a number of women who were very young girls at the time of the bombing. However, recent data on the British ankylosing spondylitis patients (Darby et al. 1985) point in the opposite direction. It is therefore indicated to reserve judgement on the applicability of the relative risk model and to continue the two important studies. Whatever the final conclusion may be, it is important to note, that present risk estimates are based on an observation period of about 30 years only and that an extension to longer times at risk could increase their values.

Are the risk estimates useful? They are hypothetical, because one can, at present, merely surmise but not prove that tumors are caused by small doses of ionizing radiations. In spite of this uncertainty, the risk estimates remain suitable for the pragmatic purposes of radiation protection. For hereditary damage and also for somatic mutations, the linear hypothesis is valid and it is therefore prudent and practicable to make a corresponding assumption also for radiation-induced tumors. The important consequence for radiation protection is, to replace the former concept of dose limits by the principle to keep radiation doses as low as reasonably achievable (ALARA).

The International Commission for Radiological Protection has attempted to formalize the ALARA principle and to develop it into a cost-benefit assessment. Some have gone to the point of assigning a monetary cost to a man sievert, which is the unit of collective dose, i.e., the sum of doses to individuals in a collective. In practice such formalistic approaches are likely to fail. The ALARA principle itself has, however, become a useful tool to reduce undesirable exposures, both in nuclear technology and in medical applications. When exposure limits are considered as ultimate ceilings, not as permissible levels, and when unnecessary exposures are avoided, average dose levels in controlled groups will stay far below the limits. This has, indeed, been achieved in nuclear industry. In medicine, similar efforts have been made, and data are now available which facilitate the optimization of diagnostic equipment and the cost-benefit assessment of diagnostic screening procedures. The controversy, in recent years, on mammography as a screening procedure exemplified the potential of the cost-benefit approach, and it has largely contributed to the reduction of the doses and to better definition of the indications for mammography. The prudent assumption of no dose threshold for somatic late effects has also helped to advance the use of modalities other than ionizing radiations.

Need for a Balanced View of Risks

The merits of the assessment system are less obvious, when it is misused, and when a philosophy is embraced which aims at total avoidance of radiation exposures or, at any rate, the complete avoidance of any "nonnatural" radiation exposure. The computation of hypothetical numbers of cancer deaths, usually in large collectives but without reference to their size, is then an effective means to generate confusion and even panic.

These problems became evident when the recent reactor accident produced contaminations in several European countries which exceeded levels legally set for the routine practice of radiation protection. Limits or derived limits were then erroneously interpreted as thresholds that separate harmless exposures from dangerous doses. On the other hand, the assumption of linearity and the risk coefficients were used to compute absolute numbers of expected cancer deaths. Even if they are formally correct, such computations can be highly misleading, when they are not related to spontaneous rates and their fluctuations due to various other factors.

For example, in a recent discussion, the claim was made that about 1000 cancer deaths would result from the collective dose of 75000 man sievert which results from the emission of $5.3 \cdot 10^{14}$ Bq of ^{14}C during the 40 years of projected operation of a reprocessing plant. The computation of the collective dose is correct. However, the statement omits the fact that more than 99.9% of this collective dose is caused after the global dispersion of ^{14}C, and over a period of several thousand years. In fact, the computed number of deaths relates to 200 generations of all of mankind. It is therefore hardly conceivable how the number 1000 could be meaningful.

Computations of assumed numbers of cancer deaths may be less widely removed from reality when applied to the consequences of large-scale radioactive contaminations from the reactor catastrophe. But they are grossly misleading when employed to induce personal anxieties. Possible increases of tumor rates in Western Europe are far smaller than the existing rates and than their fluctuations due to various controllable and uncontrollable factors. The absence of a personal thread is due to the dilution of the risk within a population of many millions. On the other hand, such dilution is no reason to disregard the possible detriments and to omit suitable measures. It is essential to distinguish between a tangible personal threat and an undesirable addition to the pool of existing detriments. To neglect risks to large populations, unless they break through the threshold of epidemiological ascertainment, would be a fatal counterposition against unfounded anxieties. Reasonable administrative measures to reduce doses, for example, from iodine-131 in milk, were therefore justified and were in line with the ALARA principle.

A more balanced view of risks and their numerical values is required. Further efforts will be needed to achieve such a view, and to have it take the place of prevailing misconceptions and collective anxieties.

References

Chmelevsky D, Kellerer AM, Spiess H, Mays CW (1986) A proportional hazards analysis of bone sarcoma rates in German ^{244}radium patients. In: Gössner W et al (eds) The radiobiology of radium and thorotrast. Urban and Schwarzenberg, München, pp 32–37

Court Brown WM, Doll R (1956) The hazards to man of nuclear and allied radiations. Report of the Medical Research Council (Br) Appendix B, p 87. Her Majesty's Stationery Office, London

Darby SC, Nakashima E, Kato H (1985) A parallel analysis of cancer mortality among atomic bomb survivors and patients with ankylosing spondylitis given X-ray therapy. JNCI 75:1–21

Ellett WH, Christy RF, Lowder WM (1985) A new dosimetry for a-bomb survivors. Radiat Prot Dosimetry 13:311–318

Failla G (1932) Radium protection. Radiology 19:12–21

Frieben A (1902) Demonstration eines Cancroids des rechten Handrückens, das sich nach langdauernder Einwirkung von Röntgenstrahlen entwickelt hatte. Fortschr Geb Röntgenstr 6:106

ICRP (1977) Annals of the ICRP, Publication 26. Recommendations of the International Commission on Radiological Protection. Pergamon, Oxford New York Frankfurt

ICRU Report 40 (1986) The quality factor in radiation protection. International Commission on Radiation Units and Measurements. Bethesda, Md

Kellerer AM, Rossi HH (1982) Biophysical aspects of radiation carcinogenesis. In: Becker FF (ed) Cancer, a comprehensive treatise. vol 1, 2nd edn. Plenum, New York, pp 569–616

Lewis EB (1957) Leukemia and ionizing radiation. Science 125:965–972

Lewis EB (1963) Leukemia, multiple myeloma, and aplastic anemia in American radiologists. Science 142:1492–1494

Loewe WE, Mendelsohn E (1981) Revised dose estimates for Hiroshima and Nagasaki. Health Phys 41:663–666

Mays CW, Spiess H, Chmelevsky D, Kellerer AM (1986) Bone sarcoma cumulative tumor rates in patients injected with ^{224}Ra. In: Gössner W et al (eds) The radiobiology of radium and thorotrast. Urban and Schwarzenberg, München, pp 27–31

Muller HJ (1927) Artificial transmutation of the gene. Science 66:84–87
National Academy of Sciences, National Research Council (1980) The effects on populations of exposure to low levels of ionizing radiation. Washington, D.C.
Rossi HH, Kellerer AM (1974) The validity of risk estimates of leukemia incidence based on Japanese data. Radiat Res 58:131–140
Rossi HH, Mays CW (1978) Leukemia risk from neutrons. Health Phys 34:353–360
Rundo J, Keane AT, Lucas HF, Schlenker RA, Stebbings JH, Stehney AF (1986) Current (1984) status of the study of ^{226}Ra and ^{228}Ra in humans at the Center for Human Radiobiology. In: Gössner W et al (eds) The radiobiology of radium and thorotrast. Urban and Schwarzenberg, München, pp 14–21
Smith PG, Doll R (1982) Mortality among patients with ankylosing spondylitis after a single course of treatment with X-rays. Br Med J 284:449–460
UNSCEAR Report (1977) Sources and effects of ionizing radiation. United Nations, General Assembly, 32nd Session, Supplement No 40 (A/32/40) UN, NY
van Kaick G, Muth H, Kaul A, Wesch H, Immich H, Liebermann D, Lorenz D, Lorenz WJ, Lührs H, Scheer KE, Wagner G, Wegener K (1986) Report on the German thorotrast study. In: Gössner W et al (eds) The radiobiology of radium and thorotrast. Urban and Schwarzenberg, München, pp 114–118
von Jagie N, Schwarz G, von Siebenrock L (1911) Blutbefunde bei Röntgenologen. Berl Klin Wochenschr 48:1220–1222
Wick RR, Chmelevsky D, Gössner W (1986) ^{224}Ra: risk to bone and haematopoietic tissue in ankylosing spondylitis patients. In: Gössner W et al (eds) The radiobiology of radium and thorotrast. Urban and Schwarzenberg, München, pp 38–44
Yoshimoto Y, Kellerer AM, Rossi HH, Nakashima E, Kato H (1981) Coordinate plots depicting basic data on members of the life span study sample. Radiation Effects Research Foundation, Research Protocol, RERF RP 10-81, 1–3

Cancer Risk from Environmental Radioactivity

W. JACOBI

Introduction

Our knowledge about sources and biological effects of ionizing radiation has been compiled and critically reviewed in the reports of UNSCEAR (1977, 1982). In recent years the radiation exposure of populations was mainly caused by natural sources and medical applications, in the latter case mainly by X-ray diagnostics. The additional dose contributions by the fallout from nuclear weapon tests or by the release of radioactive materials from nuclear power plants were negligible. This was true until the end of April 1986 when the Chernobyl accident happened.

With respect to cancer risks from environmental radioactivity, from the present point of view two problems are of main concern and will be discussed in this paper. The first part treats the lung cancer risk from inhaled short-lived decay products of radon (^{222}Rn), particularly with the radon problem in homes. In the second part, a first estimate of the dose commitment by the fallout from the Chernobyl accident is given, referring to our measurements in southern Bavaria.

Lung Cancer from Inhaled Radon Decay Products

Epidemiological Studies

Lung cancer is the oldest type of radiation-related health effect reported. As early as the beginning of the sixteenth century the so-called "Schneeberger Krankheit" was observed among underground miners in the Schneeberg-Jachimov region in Bohemia. In 1879 Haerting and Hesse diagnosed this disease as primary lung cancer. But only in the fiftieth year of this century was the real cause discovered: inhalation of the short-lived decay products ^{218}Po, ^{214}Pb, and ^{214}Bi which are built up by the decay of radon (^{222}Rn) in the air. The inhalation of these daughter atoms, which are mainly attached to dust particles, leads to a relative high alpha dose to the critical cells in the bronchial epithelium.

This suggestion was confirmed by recent epidemiological studies among different groups of Rn-exposed underground miners: uranium miners in the USA (Waxweiler et al. 1981; Whittemore et al. 1983), CSSR (Kunz et al. 1979), in Ontario/Canada (Muller et al. 1985), and France (Tirmanche et al. 1985); fluorspar miners in Newfoundland (Morrison et al. 1985); and a group of metal ore miners in Sweden (Radford et al. 1984). The results of these surveys, which involved in total nearly 30000 miners, agree with respect to the following conclusions:

1. Cancers mainly originate in the upper bronchial tree, particularly in the region of the segmental bronchi, which receives the highest alpha dose from inhaled radon daughters
2. The observed excess lung cancer rate increases nearly proportionally with the cumulative exposure to radon daughters, or the corresponding bronchial dose; only at very high exposure levels the excess risk/exposure ratio is decreasing
3. The latency period distribution of the excess lung cancer rate after irradiation is similar to the age-adjusted distribution of the normal lung cancer rate in comparable nonexposed population groups
4. The influence of nonradioactive mine dusts seems to be rather small. However, case-control studies among uranium miners in the USA and CSSR, for which smoking habits were known, indicate a synergistic influence of smoking.

These general findings are supported by the results of Rn-inhalation studies with rats (Chmelevsky et al. 1982; Chameaud et al. 1981).

In Fig. 1, the mean values (and their confidence range) of the relative excess frequency of lung cancer per unit of radon-daughter exposure are plotted as a function of the mean exposure of these groups of miners. The quantity "radon-daughter exposure" is defined as the time integral over the potential alpha-energy concentration of the radon-daughter mixture in the air inhaled by these miners during their underground work. This quantity is mostly expressed in the unit WLM (working level-months) as being 3.5 10^{-3} J h/m^3; this unit corresponds to an equilibrium-equivalent activity exposure to ^{222}Rn of 6.3 10^5 Bq h/m^3 (Rn-eq).

Except for the small group of metal ore miners in Malmberget (Sweden), the resulting relative lung cancer risk coefficients for the different groups of miners plotted

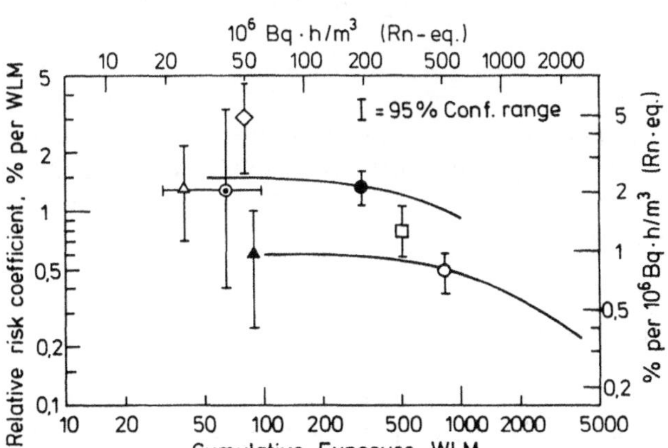

Fig. 1. Relative excess frequency of lung cancer per unit of exposure to ^{222}Rn daughters, observed in different groups of miners (in brackets, number of miners in each group). Uranium ore: ●, CSSR (2433), 1948–1975; ○, Colorado/USA (3362), 1950–1977; △, Ontario/Canada (13400), 1955–1981; ▲, (upper and lower best estimate); ⊙, France (1957), 1947–1983 (estimate). Fluorspar: □, Newfoundland/Canada (2120), 1933–1981. Iron ore: ◇, Malmberget/Sweden (1415), 1951–1976

in Fig. 1 ranges from 0.005 to 0.015 (or 0.5%–1.5%) per WLM exposure. The weighted mean value of this relative risk coefficient for miners results to:

$$r_{\text{miners}} = 0.01\ (1\%)\ \text{per WLM} \triangleq 1.6\ 10^{-8}\ \text{per Bq h/m}^3\ (\text{Rn-eq}) \quad (1)$$

The epidemiological data from miners given in Fig. 1 yield a statistically significant excess lung cancer incidence above an exposure level of 50 WLM $\triangleq$ 3 10^7 Bq h/m^3 (Rn-eq), but give no indication for a real threshold.

Proportional Hazard Model

The observed excess of lung cancer among Rn-exposed miners can be fitted rather well by a proportional hazard model (Jacobi et al. 1985; Whittemore and McMillan 1983; ICRP 1986). This model proceeds from the following basic relationship between the radiation-induced increment λ_{rad} and the normal value λ_o (without exposure) of the age-specific lung cancer rate as a function of age *t:*

$$\lambda_{\text{rad}}(t) = \lambda_o(t)\, r\, E(t-\tau) = \lambda_{o,\text{ns}}(t)\, \{1+S\}\, r\, E(t-\tau) \quad (2)$$

where $\lambda_{o,\text{ns}}$ is the age-specific rate for nonsmokers; S is an enhancement factor from smoking, averaged over the considered population group; r is the relative risk coefficient for inhaled radon daughters (see Eq. (1) and Fig. 1); and $E(t-\tau)$ is the cumulative radon-daughter exposure up to the age $(t-\tau)$. The time lag τ is refers to the minimum latency period after irradiation which is in the range of 5–10 years.

It should be emphasized that this relationship implies a multiplicative influence of smoking, and consequently an equal relative increment $\lambda_{\text{rad}}/\lambda_o$ of the radiation-induced, age-specific lung cancer rate for smokers and nonsmokers.

The integral, lifetime risk of radiation-induced lung cancer, R_{rad}, follows to

$$R_{\text{rad}} = \int_o^\infty p(t)\, \lambda_{\text{rad}}(t)\, dt \quad (3)$$

where p(t) is the survival probability from birth until age t. Taking into account the lower life expectancy of smokers, this proportional hazard model leads finally to a *relative* lifetime increment R_{rad}/R_o of lung cancer which is somewhat lower for chronic smokers than for nonsmokers.

Population Exposure to Radon Daughters

The inhalation of ^{222}Rn-decay products also yields a significant contribution to the natural radiation exposure of populations. During the past years, larger monitoring programs for radon and radon daughters in indoor air have been carried out. The results are compiled in recent reports (UNSCEAR 1982; Jacobi 1986; ICRP 1986).

These surveys have revealed that the Rn concentration in indoor air is considerably higher than in outdoor air, and varies strongly from house to house. Measured values cover a range from a few Bq/m^3 up to several 1000 Bq/m^3. For example, in the

German survey which involved about 6000 apartments, in 1% a value of more than 200 Bq/m^3 was measured; in 9 apartments the level exceeded 600 Bq/m^3 (Schmier and Wicke 1985). The mean value was about 50 Bq/m^3. In Sweden it is expected that in 1% of the houses the level might be above 800 Bq/m^3. In most houses with high Rn levels the main source is the radon influx from the underlying soil and not the radon released from building materials.

Except for the Nordic countries these surveys indicate country-averaged mean values of the ^{222}Rn concentration in indoor air in the range of 20–60 Bq/m^3. Taking into account an equilibrium factor of 0.3–0.5, this corresponds to a mean Rn-daughter concentration of 6–30 Bq/m^3, expressed in terms of the equilibrium-equivalent ^{222}Rn-concentration (EEC_{Rn}). In the UNSCEAR report (1982), a mean value of 15 Bq/m^3 (EEC_{Rn}) was assumed for the total population in the temperate regions. A similar mean value results also from the German survey.

Taking into account a mean residence probability indoors of 0.8 (approx. 7000 h per year), this would yield a mean Rn-daughter exposure of about 1 10^5 Bq h/m^3 (Rn-eq) per year, or 0.17 WLM per year. Assuming chronic exposure at this level, a cumulative mean exposure of about (7–8) 10^6 Bq/m^3 (Rn-eq) or 12–14 WLM should be expected over the whole lifetime. This is only about a factor of 5 below the exposure range at which a statistically significant excess of lung cancer has been observed among Rn-exposed miners (see Fig. 1).

Dosimetric studies indicate that under these conditions the indoor inhalation of ^{222}Rn daughters leads to a mean dose equivalent to the bronchial basal cell layer of about 15–20 mSv per year (Nuclear Energy Agency 1983). This is about a factor 10–20 times higher than the mean natural radiation exposure of other body tissues.

These recent findings make clear that more attention should be paid to the Rn problem in houses and its influence on carcinogenic effects in the lung.

Attributable Lung Cancer Risk

So far no epidemiological data from population groups living in houses with enhanced radon levels are available that would allow a direct quantitative estimate of the attributable lung cancer risk. However, an approach can be made from the described findings among Rn-exposed miners, taking into account correction factors for the different conditions in mines and houses.

In a report of the NCRP (1984), a simplifying, excess risk projection model was used to estimate the possible lifetime risk from indoor exposure to radon daughters. More reliable seem to be the risk estimates based on the previously described proportional hazard model (Jacobi and Paretzke 1985; Jacobi 1986; ICRP 1986). This type of approach is also supported by the lung cancer incidence observed among the atomic bomb survivors (Kato and Schull 1982; NIH 1985).

Figure 2 shows the relative fraction $\Delta R_{rad}/R$ of the total lifetime risk of lung cancer which should be expected on the basis of this approach for the attributable risk from chronic indoor exposure to ^{222}Rn-daughters (Jacobi 1984). It is plotted as a function of the annual exposure (upper abscissa), in WLM (1 WLM ≙ 6.3 10^5 Bq h/m^3 Rn-eq), assuming a constant exposure rate throughout the whole lifetime. On the lower abscissa, the corresponding mean concentration in indoor air is given, expressed in terms of the equilibrium-equivalent concentration of ^{222}Rn. It refers to a

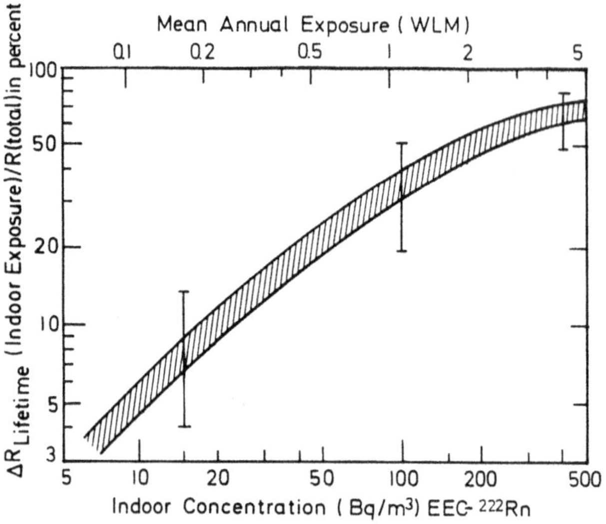

Fig. 2. Relative fraction of lifetime lung cancer risk attributable to the indoor exposure to ^{222}Rn daughters, estimated with a proportional hazard model assuming a chronic lifetime exposure at the given level. (From Jacobi 1984)

mean occupancy factor indoors of 0.8 (7000 h per year). The shadowed area indicates the variation for life expectancies of 70–80 years. Indicated are also the error ranges due to the probable uncertainty (± 50%) of the inserted relative risk coefficient *r* for the radiation-induced increment of the age-specific lung cancer rate.

It follows from this approach that in the case of a chronic exposure at the present mean indoor level of 15 Bq/m^3 (EEC) which has been measured in houses in the Federal Republic of Germany, about 8% (uncertainty range 4%–12%) of the lung cancer death rate might be associated with the indoor exposure to ^{222}Rn daughters (see Fig. 2). This relative fraction should be nearly equal for the male and female population as well as for smokers and nonsmokers, because of the multiplicative relative risk model applied. Averaged over both sexes, the mean loss of life expectancy associated with this lung cancer risk contribution results in about 10–20 days.

It should be emphasized that this risk estimate depends on the validity of the assumed linear dose-risk relationship with respect to lung cancer induced by high LET radiation. Direct epidemiological studies on this important radon problem in houses are required to test the reliability of this first estimate. Several smaller case-control studies have been started in Sweden. In a pilot study in Norway, the radon exposure in dwellings was correlated against lung cancer incidence and smoking habits data from the Norwegian cancer registry (Stranden 1986). The preliminary results support the described proportional hazard model and the conclusions derived with the approach from miners' data.

Protection Measures

The ICRP has outlined the general protection principles for limiting controllable exposures to natural sources of radiation (ICRP 1984). In this report also first guidelines for the restoration of existing buildings and the planning of future buildings are given to reach acceptable radon levels in indoor air. These recommendations have been also expressed by the German Radiation Protection Commission (SSK 1985).

In houses with high radon levels, technical countermeasures should mainly aim at a reduction of the radon influx from the underlying soil. For this purpose fairly simple methods have been developed and are applied, particularly in Sweden. Regulatory measures for the limitation of natural radioactivity in building materials seem to be not necessary (SSK 1985). One should have in mind that the radon problem in houses is only one part of the general problem of indoor air quality. Future planning of indoor air hygiene should proceed from this broader perspective.

Exposure in Southern Bavaria by the Fallout from the Chernobyl Accident

The Chernobyl accident has led to a considerable fallout of fission products in regions outside the USSR. Mainly affected were areas in Poland, the middle of Sweden

Table 1. Cumulative deposition density (A_F) of fission products in Munich–Neuherberg (GSF) after the Chernobyl accident – integrated over the time period from 29 April–8 May 1986, without correction for radioactive decay

Radio-nuclide	Radioactive half-life	A_F deposited activity kBq per m^2 soil area
Sr-89[a]	50.5 d	2.2
Sr-90[a]	29.1 a	0.21
Mo-99	66.0 h	9.6
Ru-103	39.3 d	27
Ru-106	368 d	6.9
J-129[a]	$1.57\ 10^7$ a	≤ 0.02[b]
J-131	8.04 d	92
Te-132	78.2 h	120
→ J-132	2.3 h	
J-133	20.8 h	3.7
Cs-134	2.06 a	10
Cs-136	13.1 d	4.2
Cs-137	30.0 a	19
Ba-140	12.7 d	12
→ La-140	40.3 h	
Pu-238[a]	87.7 a	$14\ 10^{-6}$
Pu-239[a]	24065 a	$40\ 10^{-6}$

[a] Only from 29 April–2 May, 1986
[b] Detection limit

and Finland, southern Bavaria, and parts of Austria and Italy. The relatively high deposition in southern Bavaria was mainly caused by a heavy rainfall with thunderstorms in the afternoon of 30 April 1986, just when the activity concentration in air had reached a maximum. The following data and exposure estimates refer to this region which involves a population of about 5 million.

Fallout Data

During the past weeks, extended measurements of relevant fission products in air, rain, soil, grass, milk and other foodstuffs have been carried out by the Institute for Radiation Protection of the GSF in Munich-Neuherberg. In addition, measurements of the β- and γ-dose rate in different areas outdoors and indoors were performed. The results have been published in a special report (GSF 1986).

In Table 1 the measured deposition densities at the location of the GSF in the north of Munich are listed. Figure 3 shows the expected decrease with time due to radioactive decay. Measurements in other parts of southern Bavaria yield fallout values which differ by a factor 0.5 to 2.5 from the data given in Table 1. Taking into account radioecological and dosimetric factors, of main concern are ^{131}J and ^{132}Te + ^{132}I in the early phase, whereas ^{137}Cs and ^{134}Cs are the determining radionuclides for the long-term exposure. The dose contribution from other radionuclides is quite small. This is also valid for ^{89}Sr, ^{90}Sr, and ^{239}Pu. It is important to note that the measured ^{137}Cs deposition of 19 kBq/m^2 is about a factor of 5 higher than the total ^{137}Cs activity per m^2 deposited in this region from all nuclear weapons tests. With respect

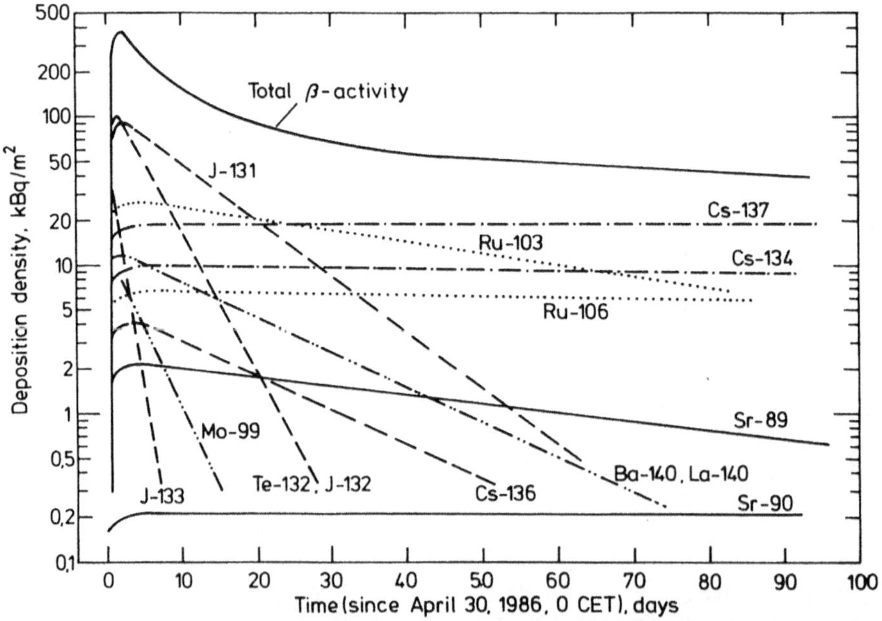

Fig. 3. Deposition density of fission products from the Chernobyl accident (measured at the location of the GSF in Neuherberg), and its decrease with time due to radioactive decay

to ^{90}Sr, this ratio is inverse: the now deposited activity is lower by a factor of 10 than the ^{90}Sr fallout from nuclear weapons tests.

For the activity transfer to man through foodchains, the activity deposited on pasture grass is one of the most important input parameters. The initial values of the activity concentration in grass in the region of Munich were in the range of 8–15 kBq/kg for ^{131}I and of 2–5 kBq/kg for ^{137}Cs. During May, a rapid growth of pasture grass occurred. This increase of biomass led to a rather strong decrease of the Cs-activity concentration in grass, with a biological half-life of 8–12 days (GSF 1986).

Transfer Through Foodchains

The most important exposure pathways are the external irradiation by the β, γ-radiation of the deposited activity, and the ingestion by the activity transfer through foodchains. Compared with these pathways, the activity intake by inhalation was small.

We have developed a specific radioecological model (ECOSYS) for the analysis of consequences of possible accidental releases from nuclear installations (Matthies et al. 1982; Pröhl et al. 1986). This model simulates the activity transfer through relevant foodchains, taking into account the seasonal variation of transfer and accumulation processes. This model has now been applied to estimate the mean activity concentration in various foodstuffs from the Chernobyl fallout as a function of time.

As an example, Fig. 4 shows the expected variation with time for ^{137}Cs, normalized to an initial deposition of 20 kBq/m^2. After a decrease during the summer months, an increase of the ^{137}Cs activity in cereal products, milk, and meat should be expected during the winter period 1986/1987. In the following years, the main source

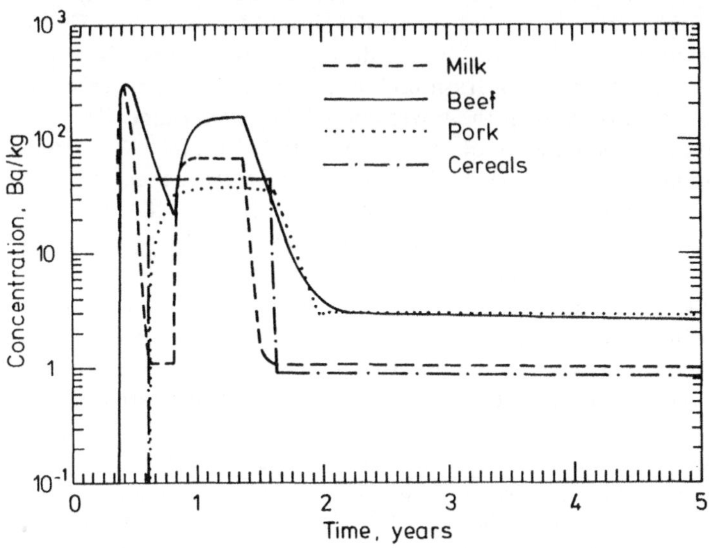

Fig. 4. Mean concentration of Cs-137 in foodstuffs as function of time, calculated with the ECOSYS model for an initial deposition density of 20 kBq/m^2; on the *abscissa,* the time since 1 January 1986, is plotted

will be the activity uptake from soil through the roots. Due to the strong fixation of cesium on soil particles, the expected activity concentration of ^{137}Cs in foodstuffs from this pathway is, however, small. This agrees with the observed transfer of ^{137}Cs from nuclear weapons tests (UNSCEAR 1977, 1982). Consequently, the human intake of ^{137}Cs and ^{134}Cs will occur mainly in the years 1986 and 1987.

Expected Dose Commitment

Applying the ECOSYS model, the activity intake with the total diet was calculated for children and adults as a function of time, referring to the fallout data listed in Table 1. The attributable dose to different tissues and the effective dose to the total body have been estimated with the dose-conversion factors recommended by ICRP (Publication 30, 1979), taking into account correction factors for children (Henrichs et al. 1985).

The additional dose contribution from external γ-radiation was determined using the Monte Carlo method (Jacob and Paretzke 1986; Jacob et al. 1986). This evaluation takes into regard the long-term decrease of the activity by run-off and migration in soil, as well as the measured mean shielding factor of buildings.

The resulting best estimates of the expected dose from the Chernobyl fallout during the first year (May 1986–April 1987) and of the dose commitment accumulated over 70 years are shown in Fig. 5 (from GSF 1986). These dose values refer to the fallout data in the region of Munich. They can be considered as representative mean values for the population in southern Bavaria. The values for the population in the northern and western parts of the Federal Republic of Germany should be considerably lower, taking into account the lower deposition densities measured in these regions.

During the first year, a dose to the thyroid of 3–12 mSv (300–1200 mrem) for children and of 0.5–2.5 mSv (50–250 mrem) for adults should be expected. The main fraction of this thyroid dose is delivered by ^{131}I during the first weeks. Taking into account the restricted consumption of fresh milk and vegetables during this period, the real thyroid dose lies probably at the lower end of the given range. This is supported by whole body measurements of the incorporated ^{131}I and ^{137}Cs activity in children from the region of Munich (Schmier and Roedler 1986); their preliminary results indicate a mean thyroid dose from ^{131}I of 2.5–3.0 mSv (250–300 mrem).

The expected dose to other tissues is considerably lower (see Fig. 5). Summing up over all exposed tissues results in an effective dose from internal and external exposure in the range of 0.5–1.5 mSv (50–150 mrem) during the first year, and a total cumulative dose during 70 years (lifetime dose, lower graph of Fig. 4) of about 1.5–6 mSv (150–600 mrem). It should be emphasized that more than one-half of this cumulative lifetime dose is received by external irradiation. The internal dose contribution is mainly due to ^{137}Cs + ^{134}Cs; compared with the dose from cesium, the expected dose contribution from ^{89}Sr and ^{90}Sr is less than one-tenth.

With respect to cesium, a comparison with the natural radionuclide ^{40}K seems suitable. For adults, the mean daily intake of ^{40}K is about 100 Bq. This leads to a total body burden of 3500–4000 Bq ^{40}K and an effective dose of 0.15–0.20 mSv (15–20 mrem) per year. Thus, the lifetime dose from ^{40}K is considerably higher than the dose by ingested ^{137}Cs + ^{134}Cs from the Chernobyl fallout.

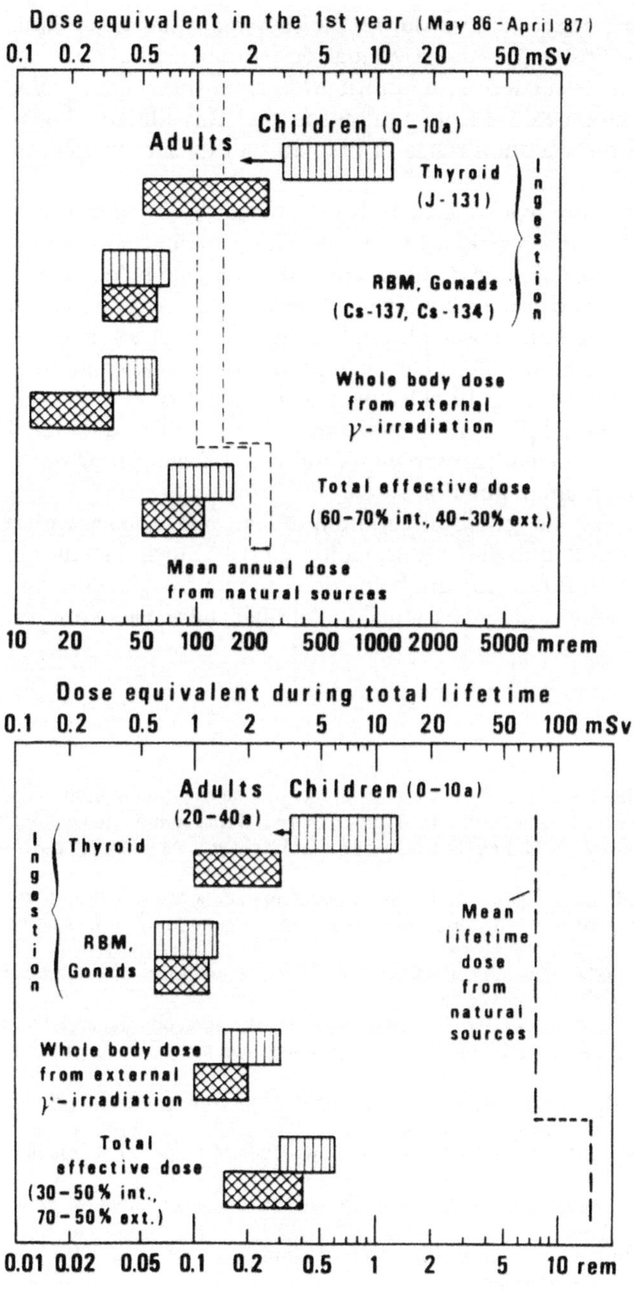

Fig. 5. Estimated dose commitment from the Chernobyl fallout (ECOSYS model), referring to the fallout data in the region of Munich. *Upper graph,* dose equivalent in the first year; *lower graph,* cumulated lifetime dose equivalent

Evaluation of Health Detriment

A first judgement of the dose commitment from the Chernobyl accident can be made by a comparison with the natural radiation exposure. For this purpose the mean values of the population exposure to natural radiation sources are plotted as dotted lines in Fig. 5. The additional effective dose during the first year after this fallout corresponds to about 30%–70% of the mean annual dose from natural sources. Integrated over 70 years, the calculated dose contribution from this fallout yields about 1%–4% of the mean lifetime dose from natural sources. This additional dose is also small compared with the variation range of the natural exposure within our population.

No epidemiological studies are available that give a statistically significant evidence of the radiation-induced cancer risk at low doses. Thus, a risk assessment at the dose levels received from the Chernobyl fallout must be based on models, extrapolating risk data which refer to considerably higher doses. For this extrapolation, usually pure linear or linear-quadratic dose-risk relationships, without a threshold, are assumed. On the basis of such models, a calculated total risk of malignant neoplasmas in the order of magnitude of 1:10000 should be expected from the Chernobyl fallout among the considered population in southern Bavaria. This additional risk is small compared with the currently observed mortality risk from cancer which is about 1:5 or 20% in the German population.

Taking into regard the local and temporal variation of cancer frequency within our population, it seems impossible to detect this additional risk. Further studies in the GSF Institute for Radiation Protection are being done to improve the dose and risk estimates from the Chernobyl accident as a function of time and age at exposure.

References

Chameaud J, Perraud R, Masse R, Lafuma J (1981) Contribution of animal experimentation in the interpretation of human epidemiological data. In: Gomez M (ed) Proceedings International Conference on Radiation Hazards in Mining, Society of Mining Engineers, New York, pp 222–227

Chmelevsky D, Kellerer AM, Lafuma J, Chameaud J (1982) Maximum likelihood estimation of the prevalence of nonlethal neoplasms – an application to radon daughter inhalation studies. Radiat Res 91:589–614

GSF, Institut für Strahlenschutz (1986) Umweltradioaktivität und Strahlenexposition in Südbayern durch den Tschernobyl-Unfall. GSF report 16/86

Henrichs K, Elsasser U, Schottola C, Kaul A (1985) Dosisfaktoren für Inhalation oder Ingestion von Radionuklidverbindungen (Altersklasse 1 Jahr, 5 Jahre). Bundesgesundheitsamt, Inst f Strahlenhygiene, ISH Hefte 78, 79

Horaček J, Plaček V, Sevč J (1977) Histological types of bronchogenic cancer in relation to different conditions of radiation exposure. Cancer 40:832–835

ICRP (1979) Limits for intakes of radionuclides by workers. ICRP Publication 30, Pergamon, Oxford

ICRP (1984) Principles for limiting exposure of the public to natural sources of radiation. ICRP Publication 39, Pergamon, Oxford

ICRP (1986) Lung cancer risk from indoor exposure to radon daughters. Report of an ICRP Task Group. Pergamon, Oxford (in preparation)

Jacob P, Paretzke HG (1986) Gamma-ray exposure from contaminated soil. Nucl Sci Eng 93:248–261

Jacob P, Paretzke HG, Rosenbaum H, Zankl M (1986) Effective dose equivalents for photon exposures from plane sources on the ground. Radiat Prot Dosimetry 14:299–310

Jacobi W (1984) Expected lung cancer risk from radon daughter exposure in dwellings. In: Proceedings International Conference on Indoor Air Quality, Stockholm, August 1984. Swedish Council for Building Research, Stockholm, pp 31–42

Jacobi W (1986) Lungenkrebs nach Bestrahlung: Das Radon-Problem. Naturwissenschaften 11: 661–668

Jacobi W, Paretzke HG (1985) Risk assessment for indoor exposure to radon daughters. Sci Total Environ 45:551–562

Jacobi W, Paretzke HG, Schindel F (1985) Lung cancer risk assessment for radon-exposed miners on the basis of a proportional hazard model. In: Stocker H (ed) Proceedings International Conference on Occupational Radiation Safety in Mining. Canadian Nuclear Association, Toronto, pp 17–24

Kato H, Schull WJ (1982) Studies of the mortality of A-bomb survivors. 7. Mortality 1950–78: Part I. Cancer mortality. Radiat Res 90:395–432

Kunz E, Sevč J, Plaček V, Horaček J (1979) Lung cancer in man in relation to different time distribution of radiation exposure. Health Phys 36:699–706

Matthies M, Eisfeld K, Müller H, Paretzke HG, Pröhl G, Wirth E (1982) Simulation des Transfers von Radionukliden in landwirtschaftlichen Nahrungsketten, GSF report S-882

Morrison HI, Semenciw RM, Mao Y, Corkill DA, Dory AB, de Villiers AJ, Stocker H, Wigle DT (1985) Lung cancer mortality and radiation exposure among the Newfoundland fluorspar miners. In: Stocker H (ed) Proceedings International Conference on Occupational Radiation Safety in Mining. Canadian Nuclear Association, Toronto, pp 365–368

Muller J, Wheeler WC, Gentleman JF, Suranyi G, Kusiak RA (1985) Study of mortality of Ontario miners. In: Stocker H (ed) Proceeding International Conference on Occupational Radiation Safety in Mining. Canadian Nuclear Association, Toronto, pp 335–343

National Council on Radiation Protection and Measurements (1984) Evaluation of occupational and environmental exposures to radon and radon daughters in the United States. NCRP Rep. No 78, Bethesda, Md

National Institutes of Health (1985) Report of the ad hoc working group to develop radioepidemiological tables. National Institutes of Health Publication No 85-2748, Washington DC

Nuclear Energy Agency (1983) Dosimetry aspects of exposure to radon and thoron daughter products. Report NEA/OECD, Paris

Pröhl G, Friedland W, Paretzke HG (1986) Intercomparison of the terrestrial food chain models FOOD-MARC and ECOSYS. GSF report 18/86

Radford EP, St Clair Renard KG (1984) Lung cancer in Swedish iron miners exposed to low doses of radon daughters. N Engl J Med 310:1485–1494

Schmier H, Roedler HD (1986) Inkorporation künstlich radioaktiver Stoffe aus dem Reaktorunfall in Tschernobyl. Mitteilungen des Instituts für Strahlenhygiene des Bundesgesundheitsamtes

Schmier H, Wicke A (1985) Results from a survey of indoor radon exposure in the Federal Republic of Germany. Sci Total Environ 45:307–310

SSK (1985) Strahlenexposition und mögliches Lungenkrebsrisiko durch Inhalation von Radon-Zerfallsprodukten. Empfehlung der Strahlenschutzkommission des BM des Inneren, 7. November 1985

Stranden E (1986) Radon-222 in Norwegian dwellings. Paper presented at the Radon Symposium of the American Chemical Society, New York, 14–16 April 1986 (in press)

Tirmanche M, Brenot J, Piechowski J, Chameaud J, Pradel J (1985) The present state of an epidemiological study of uranium miners in France. In: Stocker H (ed) Proceedings International Conference on Occupational Radiation Safety in Mining. Canadian Nuclear Association, Toronto, pp 344–349

UNSCEAR (1977) Sources and effects of ionizing radiation. United Nations, Publication No E.77.IX.1, New York

UNSCEAR (1982) Ionizing radiations: sources and biological effects. United Nations, Publication No E.82.IX.8., New York (with Annex D: Exposures to radon and thoron and their decay products)

Waxweiler RJ, Roscoe RJ, Archer VE, Thun MJ, Wagoner KJ, Lunding FE (1981) Mortality follow-up through 1977 of white underground miners cohort examined by the US Public Health Service. In: Gomez M (ed) Proceedings International Conference on Radiation Hazards in Mining. Society of Mining Engineers, New York, pp 823–830

Whittemore AS, McMillan A (1983) Lung cancer mortality among U.S. uranium miners: a reappraisal. JNCI 71:489–499

Summary of Discussion: Session 4

E. W. Hahn

Dr. Ippen was asked to comment on possible interactions between UV and chemical agents. He replied by stating that the problem is extremely complicated. Not only is light capable of changing the chemical structure of compounds, but some families of compounds have members which increase as well as others which decrease carcinogenesis. This is true, for instance, with the polycyclic aromatics. There is no means by which to predict the outcome.

Changing the topic, another attendee stated that while there was no doubt concerning the carcinogenic effects of sunlight, one should also keep in perspective that there are psychologically and physiologically beneficial effects, too. Among these would be the benefits of outdoor physical activity on the cardiovascular system, the lowering of serum cholesterol levels coincident with vitamin D synthesis, which in turn, aids in the prevention of Rickets in children and osteoporosis in the elderly, and, last but not least, the positive psychological effects of good weather and just being in sunlight. Gray dark days can certainly be depressing, as those who live in Germany know all too well. All of these are reasons why many health specialists advocate playing or just sitting in the sun. Dr. Ippen replied that of course all this is true, but that we must protect our faces and hands with light-blocking agents. This represents less than 10% of our body surface and so we can still have our vitamin D synthesis as well as the other beneficial effects mentioned.

The point was made by another attendee that while it has been clearly shown that ultraviolet radiation from sunlight does indeed induce basal and squamous cell carcinomas, the Australian and New Zealand studies found no increased risk for malignant melanoma between outdoor and indoor workers. Further, there seemed to be an important distinction between the incidence of melanoma in sunburned, untanned skin and that in carefully maintained tanned skin – where melanoma is infrequent. Dr. Ippen agreed, adding that while the relationship between light and lentigo melanoma has been established, the biggest remaining problem nevertheless is superficial spreading melanoma.

The questions was raised whether the use of UV-blocking creams has been shown to reduce the incidence of skin cancer: Dr. Ippen said several studies have shown a reduction in actinic keratosis and elastosis. Regular use of sun screens does reduce damage to the skin.

The discussion on ionizing radiation was begun by asking why, in several studies, there seems to be a decrease or a plateauing effect on carcinogenesis at the higher doses? Dr. Kellerer stated that the answer to this question is not clear-cut. One possible reason is that these plateaus and declines are actually artifacts. The data were not corrected for competing risks, such as life span shortening at the higher doses.

Dr. Jacobi added that this might explain the plateau seen in the uranium miners studies where there was a considerable shortening of lifetime due to the fact that 70% of the workers were smokers. He mentioned that another factor may come into play as well, and that is that at very high doses there is a cell-killing effect that reduces the extent of carcinogenesis.

Relevant to Dr. Kellerer's statement that at low doses the individual cell response is an all or nothing phenomenon, the following question was raised: Once the cell is hit, what are the results of such a hit – do repair mechanisms enter into the picture and does the damage then depend on the dose to the cell? Dr. Kellerer replied by emphasizing that even taking into account the complexities of cellular repair mechanisms and their dose dependence, the principle is still retained that at low doses, a cell's response is either to no dose or to an appreciable dose. Therefore, at very low doses the cellular response is postulated to be linear with dose.

The comment was made by another participant that some Scandinavian epidemiologists estimate that 10% of the lung cancers in Sweden may be caused in people living in buildings with a high background level of radon and its short-lived daughters. In view of this, the question was raised as to what the contribution of polonium-210 and lead-210 inhalation from cigarette smoke might be. The answer to that question was difficult, said Dr. Jacobi, because first the exposure from Po-210 is quite small compared with the dose from the short-lived daughters of radon and, second, there appears to be an additive or synergistic interaction between cigarette smoking and inhalation of radioactivity and induction of lung cancer. Thus, the studies show that while the relative risk for lung cancer is essentially the same for smokers and nonsmokers, the absolute risk is much greater for smokers. For instance, the Colorado uranium miners' studies have recorded about 250 cases of lung cancers to date, but only 5% of these cancers were found in the nonsmokers. As stated earlier, 70% of the miners were cigarette smokers.

The question was raised, that although there is ample evidence for the harmful effects of ionizing radiation and, indeed this conference has been emphasizing this aspect, were there any beneficial effects of low dose exposures? Dr. Jacobi replied by saying that low therapeutic doses of the order of a few hundred rads have been used quite effectively to reduce inflammatory processes, such as bursitis and certain forms of arthritis. Other studies have shown that relatively low doses to certain plant seeds can cause heterosis or an increased vigor and growth rate, and still other studies have been published which have shown that very low daily exposures have increased the life span of rodents. However, no beneficial effects, aside from radiation therapy given at higher doses, have been noted relevant to cancer. Dr. Kellerer alluded to some unpublished but recently reported data by Dr. Sheldon Wolff and his coworkers (University California, San Francisco). They found that after giving one rad of gamma radiation to lymphocytes in vitro there was a substantial decrease in chromosome breaks when the cells were subsequently exposed to higher doses. The explanation for these unusual results could not be given at this time.

Concerning the recent Chernobyl reactor accident in the Ukraine, the question was raised that in view of the fact that the levels of fallout contamination were measured and recorded and our knowledge that these isotopes can cross the placental barrier, what side effects might one expect from children born after such exposures in utero? Dr. Jacobi stated that a dose-dependent microencephaly and mental retardation and a reduction in body weight were recorded for the Japanese atomic bomb survivors. Furthermore, several studies have shown that in utero radiation from diagnostic procedures increased the incidence of leukemia. The question was then discussed whether a large-scale epidemiologic study could be started on the children born subsequent to in utero exposure to fallout from Chernobyl? Dr. Jacobi stated that even with the accepted risk factor of 1.4 for leukemia following in utero radiation, the dose from Chernobyl is likely to be so low that the probability of detecting an increased incidence of leukemia or other birth defects would be exceedingly low. A further point was made that there seemed to be sufficient evidence from in utero studies to say that the number of tumors at various sites is not enhanced, but rather accelerated, to manifest at an earlier age. Thus, high doses of in utero radiation may not be required and an epidemiologic study may very well be feasible. This conclusion was rebutted by another attendee who said that whether you get more tumors or the same number earlier may be a moot question, particularly when working with a relative risk model. Nevertheless, the consensus was that a careful evaluation should be made to determine the feasibility of such a study.

SESSION 5

Oncogenic Viruses

Chairman: E. Wecker

Viruses in Human Tumors

H. zur Hausen

Table 1 lists the possible interactions of viruses in oncogenesis and emphasizes the role of human pathogenic viruses. The majority of tumor viruses known today insert their genetic material into the host cell nucleus, where it persists. The expression of at least one viral function appears to be a prerequisite for the maintenance of the transformed state.

An interesting difference in interactions in oncogenesis is noted in infections by herpes simplex viruses. Abortive infection by these viruses modifies the host cell DNA (Schlehofer and zur Hausen 1982; Schlehofer et al. 1983). Transformation of rodent cells by these infections does not require persistence of the viral DNA. Selective DNA amplification induced by these agents may play a crucial role in transformation (Heilbronn et al. 1985). Recently it has been noted that besides herpes simplex viruses other members of the herpesvirus group, such as pseudorabies virus (B. Matz, pers. comm.) and murine cytomegaloviruses (R. Heilbronn, unpublished data), share this property. Even a member of the poxvirus group, vaccinia, is able to induce selective DNA amplification (Schlehofer et al. 1986). It remains to be seen whether this property is consistently linked to transforming functions.

A third group of agents consists of viruses causing the acquired immunodeficiency syndrome (AIDS). In this condition specific types of tumors develop as a consequence of the depressed immune function without being directly related to the AIDS virus infection.

The fourth rather interesting group includes agents suppressing oncogenicity. This property has thus far been exclusively observed in infections with autonomous or helper-dependent parvoviruses. Their mode of interaction with infected host cells may provide some clues to early events in carcinogenesis. Available evidence sug-

Table 1. Interactions of viruses with hosts and host cells in oncogenesis

	Example
Integration of the viral genome into host cell chromosomes or episomal persistence of viral DNA	Hepatitis B, papillomaviruses, EBV, HTLV1
Induction of changes analogous to chemical and physical carcinogens without persistence of viral DNA in modified cells	Herpes simplex virus, ? cytomegalovirus
Induction of immunodeficiencies, secondary development of lymphomas and Kaposi's sarcomas	HIV (AIDS)
Inhibition of oncogenesis	Parvoviruses

Table 2. Viruses involved in human oncogenesis

Epstein-Barr viruses	Burkitt's lymphoma, nasopharyngeal cancer, lymphomas in immunosuppressed individuals
Hepatitis-B virus	Primary hepatocellular carcinoma
HTLV1	Adult T-cell leukemia
HPV types 5, 8, 14, 17	Squamous cell carcinomas in patients with epidermodysplasia verruciformis
HPV types 16, 18, 31, 33, 35	Cervical cancer, vulvar cancer, penile cancer, perianal and anal cancer

gests an interference of these viruses with early events, possibly related to initiation (Heilbronn et al. 1985).

In this chapter I shall concentrate on viruses in human tumors which insert their genetic material into the host nucleus. Members of four groups of viruses have been identified thus far as playing a role in human tumors. These viruses and the respective human tumors are listed in Table 2.

The percentage of human tumors which can be linked to these infections on a worldwide scale is remarkably high. It is at present approximately 15% for both sexes (zur Hausen 1986). In females close to 20% of all cancers can be linked to viral infections, most notably cervical cancer which amounts to almost 16%. In males slightly less than 10% are virally linked, of which 6.2% represent primary hepatocellular carcinomata.

All cancers developing as a consequence of these viral infections share some characteristics, which will have to be taken into account when attempting to clarify the role of viruses in human tumors.

- they are monoclonal
- they develop only after long latency periods (in most instances after several decades, see Table 3)
- only a small percentage of infected individuals eventually develops cancer
- expression of the persisting viral genome is the rule but appears to be restricted to a specific set of genes

During the past few years the remarkable role of papilloma viruses in human cancer became evident. In particular, human anogenital cancer (including cervical, vulvar, penile, and perianal cancer) and specific rare forms of human skin cancers have been linked to these infections (see review zur Hausen and Schneider 1986). The mechanism of cancer induction following some of these infections may provide clues for the understanding of virus-linked oncogenesis in man and will be discussed in more detail subsequently.

Observations made by Rigoni-Stern and published in 1842 on the vastly different incidence of cervical cancer in prostitutes when compared to nuns mark the first important contribution to etiological factors in human genital cancer. These studies, confirmed by many subsequent analyses, stimulated research on the role of sexually transmitted agents in the genesis of this neoplasia. Up to the end of the 1960s speculations arose concerning a possible role of gonorrhea, syphilis, and trichomoniasis in

Table 3. Approximate latency periods for virus-associated human cancers

Virus	Cancer	Latency period (years)
Hepatitis B	Primary hepatocellular carcinoma	30–50
HTLV1	T-cell leukemia	30–50
Epstein-Barr	Burkitt's lymphoma	3–12
Epstein-Barr	Nasopharyngeal cancer	30–50
HPV types 5, 8, 14, 17	Skin cancer in epidermodysplasia verruciformis	3–12
HPV types 16, 18, 31, 33, 35	Cervical cancer, vulvar cancer, penile cancer, perianal and anal cancer	20–50

the induction of genital cancer, without true supportive epidemiological evidence (Rotkins 1973).

At the end of the 1960s a significant change occurred: two groups almost simultaneously reported seroepidemiological data implying an involvement of herpes simplex virus (HSV) type 2 infections in the etiology of cervical cancer (Rawls et al. 1968; Nahmias et al. 1970). During the next 10 years, in retrospective surprisingly many confirmatory manuscripts have been published, including experimental data on viral reactivation from tumor tissue, the presence of a variety of HSV-specific antigens, viral ribonucleic acid, and (much more rarely) fragments of viral DNA within premalignant and malignant tissue (reviewed in zur Hausen 1983). Since partially inactivated HSV was also shown to induce transformation of rodent cells (Duff and Rapp 1973), by the end of the 1970s HSV appeared to be a strong candidate for having a role in the induction of cervical cancer.

In 1969 my group in Würzburg attempted to implicate Epstein-Barr virus (EBV) DNA in Burkitt's lymphomas and nasopharyngeal cancer. After succeeding in the purification of EBV DNA, it was readily possible to find these genomes regularly in biopsies of both cancers by DNA–DNA or DNA–RNA hybridizations (zur Hausen and Schulte-Holthausen 1970; zur Hausen et al. 1970). Therefore it seemed obvious to use the same technology to attempt to find HSV DNA in anogenital cancer. Somewhat unexpectedly, we encountered difficulties: the analysis of a large number of biopsies provided exclusively negative results (zur Hausen et al. 1974). Early in 1972 I became convinced that HSV, if at all involved in genital cancer, could not interact with host cells in a manner analogous to other tumor virus systems known at that time, which meant leaving persisting viral DNA with partial gene expression in the transformed cell. Since another mode of interaction appeared to be unlikely at this period, and cervical cancer remained a strong candidate for a viral etiology, during 1972 we started looking for the presence of other viruses in this cancer.

There existed good reasons to select human papillomavirus (HPV) for the subsequent study: it had been known since 1907 (Ciuffo 1907) to be the causative factor of human warts. Genital warts, a particularly unpleasant infection characterized by exuberant exophytic growth, had been shown by electron microscopy to contain morphologically identical viral particles to those in common warts (Almeida et al. 1969). More importantly, there existed a substantial number of anecdotal reports, published over almost an entire century, on malignant conversion of genital warts (condylomata acuminata), usually after long duration and resistance to therapy (reviewed in zur Hausen 1977).

Wart viruses had barely been characterized at this period, mainly due to the lack of in vitro systems for viral propagation and to a remarkable host specificity (Rowson and Mahy 1967). Studies depended entirely on the availability of biopsy materials containing large quantities of viral particles. Our initial studies were performed with cRNA preparations obtained from an individual plantar wart. The first hybridization data published in 1974 (zur Hausen et al. 1974) showed that much, but by far not all, DNA from common warts hybridized with the radioactive probe. None of the genital warts and none of the cervical cancer biopsies showed a positive reaction. Since some of the genital warts analyzed contained eletron microscopically visible viral particles, this was a clear-cut suggestion that most likely different types of HPV cause condylomata acuminata. This prompted a period of analyses of individual virus particle-containing papillomas for genetic heterogeneity (Gissmann and zur Hausen 1976) and led to the identification of individual types 1 year later (Gissmann et al. 1977; Orth et al. 1977).

The identification of genital papillomavirus infections turned out to be difficult because of the low particle production in these warts. HPV6 was published in 1980 (Gissmann and zur Hausen 1980) from a rare condyloma with a high particle yield. Two new methodological approaches were of major importance for the subsequent developments: the introduction of gene cloning techniques into the papillomavirus field and the application of hybridization procedures at lowered stringency revealing the relatedness of distinct papillomavirus types, both first used in Peter Howley's laboratory (Law et al. 1979). The use of these methods led to a rapid expansion of identified types of HPVs: today 42 types have been ascertained, and most likely this number will increase further.

Gerard Orth in Paris, Stephania Jablonska in Warszau, and their colleagues identified a large number of HPV types from a rare human condition, epidermodysplasia verruciformis (Orth et al. 1980). This syndrome is characterized by an extensive verrucosis and a remarkably high rate of malignant conversions of specific types of papillomas at sun-exposed sites. It was of particular interest to find specific types of HPV, preferentially HPV5 but also HPV8 and occasionally others, within the carcinomata, although patients with epidermodysplasia verruciformis commonly reveal infections with up to 15 additional types of papillomaviruses. Cancers in this condition therefore appear to represent a fascinating example of interactions between a specific virus infection and physical carcinogens, namely the ultraviolet part of sunlight.

Returning to genital papillomavirus infections, cloning of HPV6 DNA (de Villiers et al. 1981) permitted the identification of a closely related HPV DNA, HPV11, in genital warts and laryngeal papillomas (Gissmann et al. 1982, 1983; Mounts et al. 1982). Applying conditions of low stringency hybridization, our group identified two additional types of genital papillomavirus infections, HPV16 and HPV18, by cloning their DNA directly from cervical cancer biopsies (Dürst et al. 1983; Boshart et al. 1984). Subsequently additional types have been identified, most notably HPV31 (Lorincz et al. 1985) and HPV33 (Beaudenon et al. 1986), both somewhat related to HPV16. The total number of virus types found up to now in the genital tract is 14. It appears at present that HPV6 and HPV11 are the most prevalent virus types in genital warts, accounting approximately for 90% of all condylomata acuminata and for about one-third of all oral papillomas. HPV16 and probably also HPV18 are found at external genital sites most commonly in very different lesions, characterized as bowenoid papulosis or Bowen's disease (Ikenberg et al. 1983). Histology reveals marked nuclear atypia and shows characteristics of carcinoma in situ.

All four types of HPV also infect cervical tissue. Typical papillomatous proliferations at the cervix are rare. The most common colposcopically visible lesions is represented by the "flat condyloma" (Meisels et al. 1981).

Although ardently disputed at gynecological and cytological meetings, it is likely that the histology of HPV6 and HPV11 lesions differs from that of HPV16 and HPV18 (Crum et al. 1985). The former viruses induce lesions characterized by a high degree of koilocytosis which is a pathognomonic marker for this type of infection. HPV16 and HPV18 viruses appear preferentially to induce lesions with marked nuclear atypia and a low degree or absence of visible koilocytosis. It is likely that some of the rather confusing data on the histopathology of HPV types results from infections with more than one type of HPV. Probably the majority of histopathologists would not have difficulty discriminating a bowenoid lesion from a koilocytotic condyloma at an external genital site. It would be rather surprising if the same types found in these lesions would induce a uniform histopathological pattern at cervical sites.

Kreider and his colleagues (1985) recently demonstrated that HPV11 infections induce changes characteristic of koilocytotic dysplasia upon infection of human cervical tissue heterografted beneath the renal capsule of nude mice. It is anticipated that this technique will establish the causative role of HPVs in cervical dysplasias and therefore point to an etiological role of these agents in a clearly premalignant condition. Since HPV16 and HPV18 have been directly isolated from cervical carcinoma biopsies, it is of course an important question to clarify their role in this type of cancer.

HPV16 DNA is present in approximately 50% of biopsies from cervical, vulvar, and penile cancer. It is also found in some perianal and anal cancers and in a small percentage of oral, tongue, laryngeal, and lung carcinomata. HPV18 DNA has so far only been detected in anogenital cancer where it occurs in about 20% of the biopsies tested. Approximately another 10% of these biopsies contain HPV33, HPV31, or HPV11 DNA, bringing the total proportion of biopsies with identifiable HPV types to about 80%. It is likely that the majority of additional genital tumors also contain HPV DNA of yet undefined types since bands become visible in blot hybridizations after applying conditions of lowered stringency. Therefore it appears to be justified to summarize this by stating that the majority, if not all, cervical, vulvar, and penile cancers contain HPV DNA.

In a similar manner to cancer biopsies, the majority of cervical cancer-derived cell lines tested so far contain HPV16 or HPV18 DNA, among them the well-known HeLa line (Boshart et al. 1984; Schwarz et al. 1985).

The availability of these lines and of primary cervical cancer biopsies permitted an analysis of the state of the viral DNA within the tumor cells. From the results it became evident that cell lines contain exclusively integrated viral DNA; in primary tumors integration is also regularly noted, revealing a monoclonal pattern. Some of the primary tumors have in addition episomal viral DNA (Dürst et al. 1983). Precursor lesions, bowenoid papulosis, and cervical dysplasias appear to contain preferentially nonintegrated viral DNA (Dürst et al. 1985).

The integrational pattern reveals some specificity on the viral side, opening the viral ring molecules most frequently within the E1–E2 open reading frames, thus disrupting the early region (Schwarz et al. 1985). No preferential chromosomal sites have been noted for integration (Mincheva et al. 1986). One line, Caski, contains at least 12 different integration sites in 11 distinct chromosomes.

In all cell lines analyzed thus far and in a number of primary tumors, transcription of the persisting HPV DNA has been noted. Commonly, transcripts covering the E6–E7 open reading frames are present (Schwarz et al. 1985). Some of the transcripts are fused to adjacent host cell sequences. It is not clear whether these fusion transcripts play any functional role.

Sequencing of cDNA clones of HPV18 transcripts in three cervical cancer lines revealed the existence of a small intron within the E6 open reading frame (Schneider-Gaedecke and Schwarz 1986). The second E6 exon is read in a different reading frame, resulting in a putative protein which shows some distant relationship to epidermal growth factor. It is interesting to note that the same splice donor and acceptor sites also exist in HPV16 and HPV33 DNA, but are absent in HPV6 and HPV11 DNA. It remains to be seen whether this has any functional significance.

The regularity of transcription in HPV-positive cervical cancer cells and the consistent expression of the E6–E7 open reading frames suggest a role of this genetic activity in the maintenance of the transformed state. Integration of viral DNA within E1–E2 with a likely disruption of an intragenomic regulation may represent another event important for malignant conversion. Recently some still somewhat preliminary studies further emphasized the role of HPV expression in the maintenance of the malignant phenotype. Stanbridge and his coworkers (1982) demonstrated that fusion of HeLa cells to normal human fibroblasts or keratinocytes results in a suppression of the malignant phenotype. Loss of chromosomes from the nontransformed donor, apparently in particular chromosome no. 11, leads to a reacquisition of malignant growth upon heterotransplantation into nude mice. Since HeLa cells express HPV18 RNA, it was clearly interesting to analyze HPV18 expression in the nonmalignant HeLa hybrids as well as in their malignant revertants.

The data obtained thus far (Schwarz et al., to be published) indicate that no difference occurs in HPV18 expression in HeLa cells, their hybrids with normal cells, or in malignant revertants upon cultivation of these cells in tissue culture. Under these conditions also no differences are noted in clonability and growth in soft agar. Whereas HeLa cells and malignant revertants continued to express HPV18 DNA after transplantation into nude mice, initial experiments suggested a complete block of HPV18 expression in the nonmalignant hybrid lines. Although these data were difficult to interpret due to the invasion of murine cells into these chambers, these and more recent studies, using differentiation-inducing chemicals in vitro, suggest a control of HPV expression at the transcriptional level in nontumorigenic hybrid cells.

The interpretation of these data is schematically outlined in Fig. 1. The data point to an intracellular control of HPV expression by cellular genes. These genes most likely are modified and functionally inactive in HeLa cells but are contributed to the

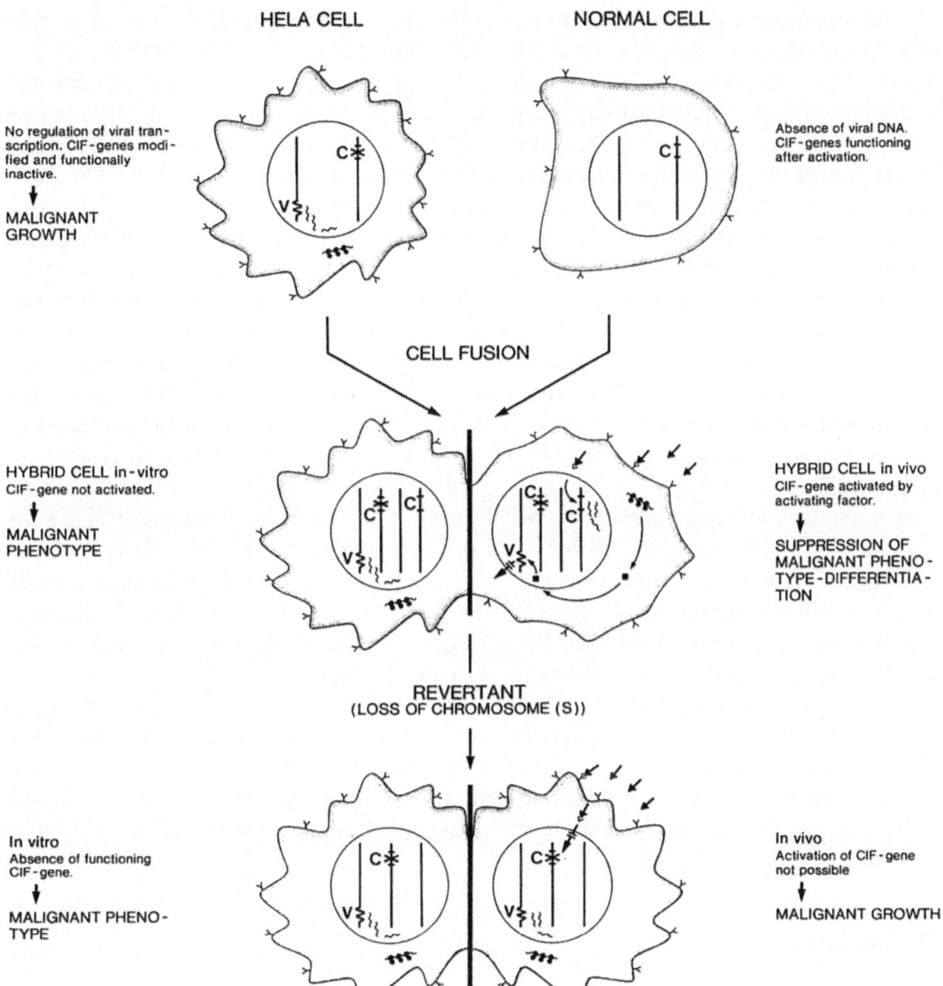

Fig. 1

hybrids by the normal donor. Obviously, they are not expressed in tissue culture, but seem to require activation by a putative humoral factor. This occurs upon heterotransplantation to the nude mouse.

These data, if confirmed for other human tumor cell lines, support a concept viewing the development of human cancer as a failing host-cell control of persisting viral genes (zur Hausen 1977, 1980, 1986). The model derived therefrom can readily explain the frequently observed synergism between papillomavirus infections and initiating events (zur Hausen 1983b). Initiators should interact by modifying cellular control functions or the binding sites recognized by the cellular suppressing factor within the viral genome.

Factors modifying cellular genes in the development of genital cancer are at present poorly defined. Smoking, viral infections with initiating properties (e.g., herpes simplex virus and cytomegalovirus), and potentially mutagenic metabolites in chronic inflammations should be particular risks for cervical sites and are probably much less active at external genital sites (zur Hausen 1983b). This could account for the much higher risk of cervical cancer in comparison to vulvar and penile cancer and for a different age distribution of the latter in comparison to cancer of the cervix.

The data suggest the existence of an intracellular surveillance mechanism which controls papillomavirus infections. It may have far-reaching implications for other human tumor virus infections as well, possibly controlled by a similar mechanism. This could represent an ancestral defense mechanism, preceding immunological control functions, protecting the host at the cellular level against potentially lethal functions of coevolving viruses. The expression of these viral functions in differentiating cells which are unable to proliferate, permitting new replication and maturation of the respective papillomaviruses, points to a fine tuning of host–virus and virus–host adaptations.

Cancer as a result of failing host-cell control of persisting viral genes could readily explain the long latency periods between primary infections of cancer-linked viruses and tumor appearance. It also provides a convenient explanation why only a small number of infected individuals develops the respective cancer type. As in addition to a persisting viral genome modificaitons in both alleles of suppressing genes are required, monoclonality of the arising tumor can be predicted.

The concept developed here offers a new view for understanding the etiology of smoking-related cancers. Increasingly, HPV genomes have been demonstrated in some of them (zur Hausen 1986). If such tumors arise from a similar interaction between persisting viral infections and smoking-related chemical carcinogens, new strategies can be developed for the control and therapy of these common human cancers.

References

Almeida JD, Oricl JD, Stannard LM (1969) Characterization of the virus found in human genital warts. Microbios 3:225–229

Beaudenon S, Kremsdorf D, Croissant O, Jablonska S, Wain-Hobson S, Orth G (1986) A novel type of human papillomavirus associated with genital neoplasias. Nature 321:246–249

Boshart M, Gissmann L, Ikenberg H, Keinheinz A, Scheurlen W, zur Hausen H (1984) A new type of papillomavirus DNA, its presence in genital cancer biopsies and in cell lines derived from cervical cancer. EMBO J 3:1151–1157

Ciuffo G (1907) Innesto positivo con filtrato di verruca vulgare. Giorn Ital Mal Venereol 48:12–17

Crum CP, Mitao M, Levine RU, Silverstein S (1985) Cervical papillomaviruses segregate within morphologically distinct precancerous lesions. J Virol 54:675–681

de Villiers E-M, Gissmann L, zur Hausen H (1981) Molecular cloning of viral DNA from human genital warts. J Virol 40:932–935

Dürst M, Gissmann L, Ikenberg H, zur Hausen H (1983) A papillomavirus DNA from a cervical carcinoma and its prevalence in cancer biopsy samples from different geographic regions. Proc Natlo Acad Sci USA 80:3812–3815

Dürst M, Kleinheinz A, Hotz M, Gissmann L (1985) The physical state of human papillomavirus type 16 DNA in benign and malignant genital tumors. J Gen Virol 66:1515–1522

Duff R, Rapp F (1973) Oncogenic transformation of hamster embryo cells after exposure to inactivated herpes simplex virus type I. J Virol 12:209–217

Gissmann L, zur Hausen H (1976) Human papillomaviruses: physical mapping and genetic heterogeneity. Proc Natl Acad Sci USA 73: 1310–1313
Gissmann L, zur Hausen H (1980) Partial characterization of viral DNA from human genital warts (condylomata acuminata). Int J Cancer 25: 605–609
Gissmann L, Pfister H, zur Hausen H (1977) Human papillomaviruses (HPV): characterization of four different isolates. Virology 76: 569–580
Gissmann L, Diehl V, Schulz-Coulon H, zur Hausen H (1982) Molecular cloning and characterization of human papillomavirus DNA from a laryngeal papilloma. J Virol 44: 393–400
Gissmann L, Wolnik H, Ikenberg H, Koldovsky U, Schnürch HG, zur Hausen H (1983) Human papillomavirus types 6 and 11 sequences in genital and laryngeal papillomas and in some cervical cancer biopsies. Proc Natl Acad Sci USA 80: 560–563
Heilbronn R, Schlehofer JR, Yalkinoglu AÖ, zur Hausen H (1985) Selective DNA amplification induced by carcinogens (initiators): evidence for a role of proteases and DNA polymerase alpha. Int J Cancer 36: 85–91
Ikenberg H, Gissmann L, Gross G, Grussendorf-Conen E-I, zur Hausen H (1983) Human papillomavirus type 16 related DNA in genital Bowen's disease and in bowenoid papulosis. Int J Cancer 32: 563–565
Kreider JW, Howett MK, Wolfe SA, Bartlett GL, Zaino RJ, Sedlacek TV, Mortel L (1985) Morphological transformation in vivo of human uterine cervix with papillomavirus from condylomata acuminata. Nature 317: 639–641
Law MF, Lancaster WD, Howley PM (1979) Conserved polynucleotide sequences among the genomes of papillomaviruses. J Virol 32: 199–211
Lorincz AT, Lancaster WD, Temple GF (1985) Detection and characterization of a new type of human papillomavirus. J Cell Biochem [Suppl] 9c: 75
Meisels A, Roy M, Fortier M, Morin C, Casas-Cordero M, Shah KV, Turgeon H (1981) Human papillomavirus infection of the cervix: the atypical condyloma. Acta Cytol 25: 7–16
Mincheva A, Gissmann L, zur Hausen H (1986) Chromosomal integration sites of human papillomavirus DNA in three cervical cancer cell lines mapped by in-situ hybridization. (Submitted for publication)
Mounts P, Shah KV, Kashima H (1982) Viral etiology of juvenile and adult onset squamous papilloma of the larynx. Proc Natl Acad Sci USA 79: 5425–5429
Nahmias AJ, Josey WE, Naib ZM, Luce CF, Guest BA (1970) Antibodies to herpes virus hominis types I and II in humans: II. Women with cervical cancer. Am J Epidemiol 91: 547–552
Orth G, Favre M, Croissant O (1977) Characterization of a new type of human papillomavirus that causes skin warts. J Virol 24: 108–120
Orth G, Favre M, Breitburd F, Croissant O, Jablonska S, Obalek S, Jarzabek-Chorzelska M, Rzesa G (1980) Epidermodysplasia verruciformis: a model for the role of papillomaviruses in human cancer. In: Essex M, Todaro G, zur Hausen H (eds) Viruses in naturally occurring cancers. Cold Spring Harbor, NY, pp 259–282
Rawls WE, Tompkins WAF, Figueroa ME, Melnick JL (1968) Herpes simplex virus type 2: association with carcinoma of the cervix. Science 161: 1255–1256
Rigoni-Itern D (1842) Fatti statistici relativi alle malattie cancrose. Giornale Service Progr Pathol Terap Ser 2: 507–517
Rotkins ID (1973) A comparison review of key epidemiological studies in cervical cancer related to current searches for transmissible agents. Cancer Res 33: 1353–1367
Rowson KEK, Mahy BWJ (1967) Human papova (wart) virus. Bacteriol Rev 31: 110–131
Schlehofer JR, zur Hausen H (1982) Induction of mutations within the host cell genome by partially inactivated herpes simplex virus type 1. Virology 122: 471–475
Schlehofer JR, Gissmann L, Matz B, zur Hausen H (1983) Herpes simplex virus induced amplification of SV 40 sequences in transformed Chinese hamster cells. Int J Cancer 32: 99–103
Schlehofer JR, Ehrbar M, zur Hausen H (1986) Vaccinia virus, herpes simplex virus and carcinogens induce DNA amplification in a human cell line and support replication of a helper-dependent parvovirus. Virology 152: 110–117
Schneider-Gaedicke A, Schwarz E (1986) Different human cervical carcinoma cell lines show similar transcription patterns of human papillomavirus type 18 genes. EMBO J 5: 2285–2292
Schwarz E, Freese UK, Gissmann L, Mayer W, Roggenbuck B, zur Hausen H (1985) Structure and transcription of human papillomavirus sequences in cervical carcinoma cells. Nature 314: 111–114

Stanbridge EJ, Der CJ, Doersen C-J, Nishimi RY, Peehl DM, Weissman BE, Wilkinson JE (1982) Human cell hybrids: analysis of transformation and tumorigenicity. Science 215:252–259
zur Hausen H (1977a) Human papillomaviruses and their possible role in squamous cell carcinomas. Curr Top Microbiol Immunol 78:1–30
zur Hausen H (1977b) Cell-virus gene balance hypothesis of carcinogenesis. Behring Inst Mitt 61: 23–30
zur Hausen H (1980) The role of viruses in human tumors. Adv Cancer Res 33:77–107
zur Hausen H (1982) Human genital cancer: synergism between two virus infections or synergism between a virus infection and initiating events. Lancet 2:1370–1373
zur Hausen H (1983) Herpes simplex virus in human genital cancer. Int Rev Exp Pathol 25:307–326
zur Hausen H (1986) Intracellular surveillance of persisting viral infections: human genital cancer resulting from a failing cellular control of papilloma-virus gene expression. Lancet 2:489–491
zur Hausen H, Schneider A (1986) The role of papillomaviruses in human anogenital cancer. In: Howley PM, Salzman NP (eds) The papovaviridae, the papillomaviruses. Plenum, New York (to be published)
zur Hausen H, Schulte-Holthausen H (1970) Presence of EB virus nucleic acid homology in a "virus-free" line of Burkitt tumor cells. Nature 227:245–248
zur Hausen H, Schulte-Holthausen H, Klein G, Henle W, Henle G, Chifford P, Santesson L (1970) EBV DNA in Burkitt tumours and anaplastic carcinomas of the nasopharynx. Nature 228:1056–1058
zur Hausen H, Meinhof W, Scheiber W, Bornkamm GW (1974) Attempts to detect virus specific DNA sequences in human tumors: I. Nucleic acid hybridizations with complementary RNA of human wart virus. Int J Cancer 13:650–656

Strategies in the Prevention of Infections by Oncogenic Viruses

F. Deinhardt

Introduction

Viruses of various families of the RNA or the DNA viruses are associated with tumors in both animals and man. The mechanisms by which such oncogenic viruses transform normal cells into malignant cells differ. However, they all produce genetic changes and/or changes in the expression of genes which are responsible for controlling normal or abnormal cellular functions. Simply put, a strategy to prevent infection with oncogenic viruses (or rather, to prevent the oncogenic result of such infection) would be to interfere with viral replication, by inhibiting integration of the viral genome into the host-cell genome, or by suppression of viral gene expression, each of which can lead to genetic alteration in host cells. Inhibition of viral replication, at least in some experimental systems, has been achieved by blocking viral enzymes through providing synthetic small substrate decoys in large excess. Blocking the reverse transcriptase of retroviruses with various chemical substances also has been tried in many studies. However, although chemicals which preferentially block viral reverse transcriptases and not host-cell enzymes have been identified, their therapeutic efficiency has been disappointing. This is because they only inhibit virus multiplication but do not eliminate the already integrated viral genomes. Also, such chemicals would have to be given for a long time, possibly even lifelong, which is impracticable and in most cases impossible because of toxicity.

Immunological elimination of virus-infected normal or transformed cells is an effective defense mechanism. Such cells usually persist only when the mechanism fails because the infected and/or transformed cells do not express neoantigens which are recognized by the immunological surveillance system or because the immune surveillance is deficient. A classical example of such deficiency is the destruction of key cells of the surveillance system by infection with retroviruses, i.e., the infection and lysis of T-helper cells by LAV/HTLV III or as recently renamed, HIV (Coffin et al. 1986).

Other approaches could be the blocking of receptor sites on target cells, use of exogenous interferon, or induction of interferon production in the host. Some encouraging results have been obtained in the interferon treatment of herpes virus infections, papovavirus-induced tumors, and hepatitis B, but this approach cannot be considered successful as a routine therapy (Dunk et al. 1986). In addition, although interferon can be given for a short period, to prevent spread of infection in the face of an epidemic, it would be impossible to use interferon lifelong, to protect individuals from potentially oncogenic viruses which may infect at any time. It is clear, therefore, that prevention of infection over prolonged periods of time would be the most effective approach to controlling oncogenic viruses, as it also is for most other infections and particularly for viruses. Thus, the remainder of my paper focuses only on prevention, and I will draw in more detail on the control of one particular oncogenic virus, hepatitis B virus (HBV), by vaccination – an area in which we have come a long way towards success – and a couple of other oncogenic viruses.

Strategies of Prevention of Infection: General Considerations

Infection can be prevented by interruption of the chain of transmission of a particular virus, or through passive or active immunization. These strategies are effective for horizontally transmitted viruses, but usually fail with vertically transmitted, endogenous viruses, a particularly frequent situation in experimental retrovirus systems (Klein 1980). Little or nothing can prevent persistence of this type of infection in random outbred human populations, short of ethically unacceptable, forced sterilization of infected individuals.

In contrast, public health measures and immunization can be most efficient in controlling horizontally transmitted disease. Viruses transmitted by animal vectors or those with other host species in addition to man can be controlled through the vector, or attempts can be made to eliminate the virus in the respective animal host species. For example, rabies (although not an oncogenic virus) is controlled by eliminating rabid animals and through animal immunization against rabies. Control of those virus infections transmitted by direct contact, particularly through intimate contact, is difficult, particularly when the period of infectivity extends beyond the period of clinical disease. Epstein-Barr virus (EBV), HBV and the retroviruses HTLV I, HTLV II, and LAV/HTLV III (HIV) belong to this group.

Prevention of Infection with Specific Viruses

Immunization Against Epstein-Barr Virus

Active immunization appears to be the only effective way of controlling EBV infections and their occasional associations with later lymphomatous diseases or nasopharyngeal carcinoma. Attenuated live virus vaccines of the conventional type are impracticable because it is impossible to test such virus strains for stable loss of their oncogenic potential for man.

In the past, production of killed virus vaccines, containing inactivated whole virus or split virus, was also impracticable, because we lacked culture systems yielding sufficient amounts of virus for vaccine production. However, identification of the EBV membrane antigen gp 340 as an immunogen inducing neutralizing, protective antibodies in nonhuman primates was a major step towards the development of an EBV subunit vaccine. It has been shown that although 50% of gp 340 consists of carbohydrate, specific antibodies appear to bind to the protein and not to the sugar (Morgan et al. 1984). The part of the EBV genome coding for gp 340 has been identified (Hummel et al. 1984), sequenced (Biggin et al. 1984), and cloned, and expression of these clones in bacterial, yeast, or mammalian cells has given encouraging results, meaning that in future, genetic engineering techniques can produce the protein part of gp 340 as an immunogen.

The use of hybrid viruses, such as vaccinia virus carrying the gene for EBV gp 340, for producing the antigen in cell-culture systems, or as a hybrid virus vaccine used directly in man is also being considered, but the well-known adverse reactions of vaccinia virus in man and the rather poor immune response of such hybrid vaccines in animal trials make the latter approach rather questionable. Nevertheless, the results with gp 340 purified from EBV give cause for some optimism, as recently expressed by Epstein:

> A vaccine derived from the high molecular weight glycoprotein (gp 340) component of the Epstein-Barr (EB) virus membrane antigen conferred complete protection against a 100% lymphomagenic dose of EB virus in the cottontop tamarin, the animal of choice for experiments with EB virus. The membrane antigen gene has already been cloned, and the development of a vaccine for use in man should now be possible. Such a vaccine could be tested first against infectious mononucleosis, because the effectiveness of vaccination would become evident in a relatively short time. Field trials against Burkitt's lymphoma and nasopharyngeal cancer could follow. (Epstein 1986)

Public Health Measures and Immunization Against Retroviruses

Infection by horizontally transmitted retroviruses, such as HIV, can be limited by public health measures and education of risk groups about the modes of transmission of these viruses (Infectious Disease Society of America 1986; WHO 1986). In addition, major efforts are underway to develop vaccines for active immunization against these retroviruses, but variability of the viral envelope antigens which induce the production of neutralizing antibodies makes this particularly difficult. Even so, it is hoped that conserved antigenic epitopes will be found to overcome this problem (Starcich et al. 1986; Sarma and Gruber 1986; Newman et al. 1986; Rasheed et al. 1986).

Immunization Against Papovaviruses

Immunization against papovaviruses is even further away but identification of the association of particular papovaviruses with specific neoplasias in man and the detailed characterization of these viruses may also open ways for vaccine development. In the meantime, some encouraging results have been obtained with treating at least some of the conditions caused by papovaviruses (i.e., papillomas) with interferons.

Immunization Against Hepatitis B Virus

Of all the human viruses with oncogenic potential, the greatest advance has been made towards the control of HBV, which is at least one of the causes of hepatocellular carcinoma (HCC; Robinson et al. 1984). Chronic HBV infection is associated with HCC: epidemiological evidence has shown that at least in some populations the chance of developing HCC is more than 160 times greater in HBV carriers than in HBV-free individuals (Beasley and Hwang 1984).

HBV-DNA has been shown to be integrated into the genome of cells of many HCC (Edman et al. 1980; Brechot et al. 1980; Chakraborty et al. 1980; Fowler et al. 1986), and most recently transacting gene activity in HBV has been demonstrated (Jameel and Siddiqui 1986; Zahm and Hofschneider, personal communication). However, particularly in European and North American countries, not all cases of HCC occur in HBV carriers, and other causes such as alcohol must also be considered (Bassendine 1986; Fowler et al. 1986). In developing countries, particularly in Africa and Asia, HCC is probably caused by two events, i.e., HBV infection in conjunction with another carcinogen, for example, aflatoxins. However, it has been shown that woodchuck hepatitis virus, a virus belonging to the same group as HBV, the hepadna (hepatitis DNA) viruses, causes HCC in woodchucks held under experimental conditions free of contact to other carcinogens (Purcell, Tenant and Popper, personal communication).

Although understanding the precise pathogenesis of HCC may still take a long time, preventing the HBV carrier state should at least substantially reduce the incidence of HCC in most areas of the world. HBV is prevalent in populations with a high incidence of HCC, and in these populations HBV infection usually occurs very early in life, either perinatally or during the first years of infancy. Unfortunately, as compared with infection occurring later in life, these infections have a greater tendency to lead to HBV carrier states with chronic hepatitis, cirrhosis, and/or development of HCC.

Whereas transmission of HBV by blood (and blood products) or unsterilized needles (or other equipment penetrating the skin) can be avoided by proper hygienic techniques, education of drug addicts, and screening of blood donors for HBV, transmission by intimate contact or perinatal infection can only be prevented through immunization. Although HBV has not been grown in cell or tissue cultures and can only be transmitted to man and apes, especially chimpanzees, the virus has been fully characterized, the genome and most of its gene products have been identified, and the genome has been cloned, sequenced, and expressed in bacterial, yeast, and mammalian cells (Gerber and Thung 1985; Seeger et al. 1986).

Vaccines were produced first from HBsAg present in vast excess in the blood plasma of HBV carriers (Hilleman et al. 1978; Stevens et al. 1984; Deinhardt and Zuckerman 1985). These vaccines consisted of highly purified HBsAg and incorporation of several inactivation steps in their production process guaranteed absence of any infectious agents. Nevertheless, apprehension about the then unknown etiology of acquired immunodeficiency disease (AIDS) hampered the acceptance of this vaccine. In addition, the vaccine was and still is expensive, so other ways of HBV vaccine production were explored.

Expression of HBsAg from cloned HBV-DNA in bacterial, yeast, or mammalian cells, and the construction of hybrid viruses, such as vaccinia virus carrying that part of the HBV genome coding for HBsAg were two approaches (Hilleman 1985; Moss et al. 1984; Purcell and Gerin 1985; Scolnick et al. 1984; Zuckerman 1985). Vaccines prepared from HBsAg produced in yeast cells have been developed by several groups; they have been evaluated already in large clinical studies in man and are ready for general use (Hilleman et al. 1984; McAleer et al. 1984; Scolnick et al. 1984). The immune responses to either vaccine, the human plasma-derived or the recombinant, have been equally effective, resulting in 80%–99% seroconversion in healthy adults

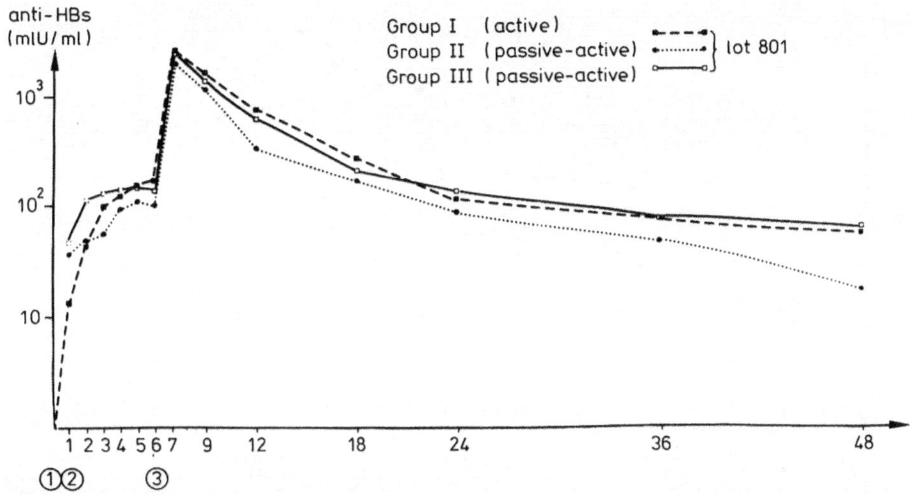

Fig. 1. Comparison of active and passive-active immunization with plasma-derived hepatitis B vaccine (H-B-Vax, Merck Sharp & Dohme)

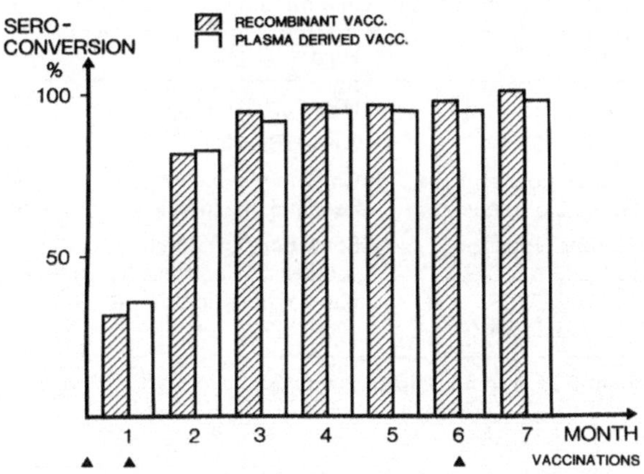

Fig. 2. Seroconversion rates (anti-HBs) after vaccination with plasma-derived (H-B-Vax) or recombinant (Merck Sharp & Dohme) hepatitis B vaccine

or newborns. Side reactions have been minimal and in cases where immediate protection was needed, passive-active immunization by simultaneously inoculating hepatitis B immunoglobulin (HBIG) and vaccine proved highly effective, inducing an immediate passive immunity without interfering with the development of active immunity (Zachoval et al. 1984). Comparison of passive-active immunization with active immunization alone with the plasma-derived vaccine is given in Fig. 1 and a comparison of active immunization with the plasma-derived or recombinant vaccine in Fig. 2 and 3. As can be seen, active or passive-active immunization have the same long-term effect and there is no statistically significant difference between the plasma-derived and the recombinant vaccines. Similar results were obtained in other studies, both in adults and in newborns (Beasley et al. 1983; Goudeau et al. 1983; Kanai et al. 1985; Kwang-Juei et al. 1985; Zanetti et al. 1986). Recently, the possi-

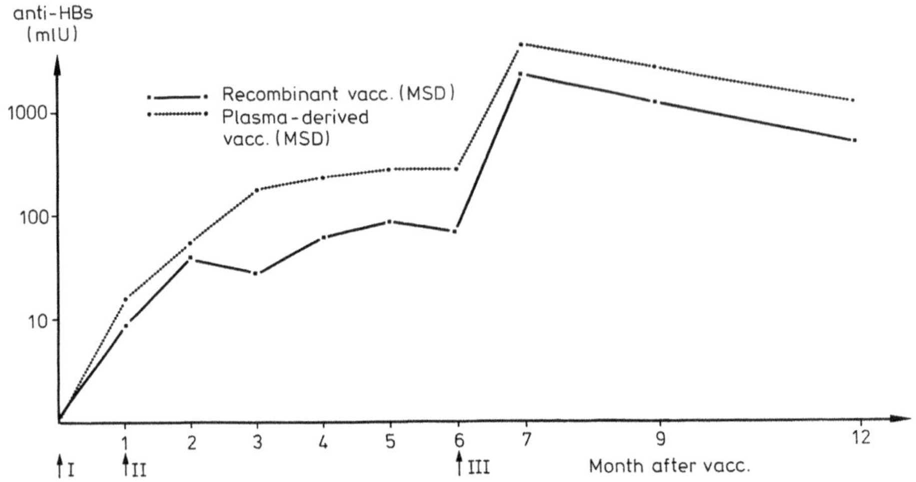

Fig. 3. Anti-HBs after active immunization of healthy young adults with recombinant hepatitis B vaccine and plasma-derived hepatitis B vaccine (geometric mean of anti-HBs concentration)

Table 1. Patterns of hepatitis B prevalence. (Modified from Deinhardt and Gust 1982)

Low	Intermediate	High
HBsAg, 0.2%–0.5%	HBsAg, 2%–7%	HBsAg, 8%–20% [a]
Anti-HBs, 4%–6%	Anti-HBs, 20%–55%	Anti-HBs, 70%–95%
Childhood infection, infrequent	Childhood infection frequent, neonatal infection frequent	Childhood infection highly frequent, neonatal infection highly frequent
Australia, Central Europe, North America	Eastern Europe, Japan, Mediterranean, southwest Asia, USSR, parts of the Middle East	Some parts of China, southern Asia, tropical Africa, parts of the Middle East

[a] Prevalences up to 50% have been identified in some isolated Pacific islands

bility that even more immunogenic HBV vaccines could be prepared by including the pre-S gene products in vaccine formulations has been discussed, but this question needs further study. It is, however, possible to produce recombinant or even synthetic vaccines containing both the antigenic epitopes of the HBsAg and the pre-S region (Heerman et al. 1984; Milich et al. 1985; Neurath et al. 1985; Offensperger et al. 1985; Klinkert et al. 1986).

The use of such vaccines in various regions of the world depends on the prevalence of HBV in the population groups there. An expert group of the World Health Organization (WHO) has defined areas of low, intermediate, and high prevalence of hepatitis B (as given in Table 1) and has recommended strategies of vaccination depending on the prevalence of HBV in the region (Table 2; Deinhardt and Gust 1982). Hepatitis B virus infects man and has no known animal vectors; therefore, a vaccination program could eliminate HBV infections and result at least in a substantial reduction in the occurrence of HCC, one of the 10 most frequent cancers

Table 2. Recommendations for hepatitis B vaccine prophylaxis according to prevalence of HBV. (Modified from Deinhardt and Gust 1982)

Low prevalence		Intermediate or high prevalence	
Preexposure	Postexposure	Pre-exposure[a]	Post-exposure[a]
High risk groups (health care personnel, dialysis patients, institutionalized patients, drug addicts, male homosexuals, military recruits, prostitutes)	Accidental percutaneous exposure, infants of HBsAg-positive mothers, sexual contacts of acute cases, and carriers	All infants	Infants of HBsAg-positive mothers

[a] Ideally infants of all mothers, but this may depend on availability of vaccine

worldwide. However, many organizational and financial restrictions must be overcome before a worldwide hepatitis B vaccine program can become effective. Development of less expensive vaccines, transfer of technologies to the developing countries where the vaccine is needed most and where the vaccine could be produced less expensively, as well as the organization of international pilot or demonstration projects with the help of WHO are some of the efforts now being undertaken to reduce in particular the perinatal and early childhood infection in the intermediate and high prevalence areas. It is obvious that double-blind, placebo-controlled studies cannot be conducted to see whether the incidence of HCC in 10–20 years time in a vaccinated group is lower than in controls. However, it can be shown which vaccination schedules give optimal protection from HBV infection, and as vaccination cannot begin in all areas of a given region at once, a difference in the time of decline of HCC related to the time when vaccination was started should be observed, and this situation will give us additional data about the role of chronic HBV infections in the pathogenesis of HCC.

In this sense, the HBV vaccine is important not only for preventing a disease of major public health importance, resulting frequently in prolonged illness, sometimes fulminant fatal disease, and leading in some cases (approx. 5%–30%) to chronic debilitating hepatitis and cirrhosis, but because it is the first vaccine preventing or at least reducing the incidence of a frequent human neoplasia, namely HCC.

References

Bassendine MF (1986) Alcohol – a major risk factor for hepatocellular carcinoma? J Hepatol 2: 513–519

Beasley RP, Hwang LY (1984) Epidemiology of hepatocellular carcinoma. In: Vyas GN, Dienstag JL, Hoofnagle JH (eds) Viral hepatitis and liver disease. Grune and Stratton, Orlando, pp 209–224

Beasley RP, Hwang LY, Lee GGY, Lan CC, Roan CH, Huang FY (1983) Prevention of perinatally transmitted hepatitis B virus infection with hepatitis B vaccine. Lancet 2:1099–1102

Biggin M, Farrell PJ, Barrell BG (1984) Transcription and DNA sequence of the *Bam* HI L fragment of B95-8 Epstein-Barr virus. EMBO J 3:1083–1090
Brechot C, Pourcel C, Louise A, Rain B, Tiollais P (1980) Presence of integrated hepatitis B virus DNA sequences in cellular DNA of human hepatocellular carcinoma. Nature 286:533–535
Chakraborty PR, Ruiz-Opazo N, Shouval D, Shafritz DA (1980) Identification of integrated hepatitis B virus DNA and expression of viral RNA in an HBsAg-producing human hepatocellular carcinoma cell line. Nature 286:531–533
Coffin J, Haase A, Levy JA, Montagnier L, Oroszlan S, Teich N, Temin H, Toyoshima K, Varmus H, Vogt P, Weiss R (1986) What to call the AIDS virus? Nature 321:10
Deinhardt F, Gust ID (1982) Viral hepatitis. Bull WHO 60:661–691
Deinhardt F, Zuckerman AJ (1985) Immunization against hepatitis B: report on a WHO meeting on viral hepatitis in Europe. J Med Virol 17:209–217
Dunk AA, Ikeda T, Pignatelli M, Thomas HC (1986) Human lymphoblastoid interferon. In vitro and in vivo studies in hepatocellular carcinoma. J Hepatol 2:419–429
Edman JC, Gray P, Valenzuela P, Rall LB, Rutter WJ (1980) Integration of hepatitis B virus sequences and their expression in a human hepatoma cell. Nature 286:535–538
Epstein MA (1986) Vaccination against Epstein-Barr virus: current progress and future strategies. Lancet 1:1425–1427
Fowler MJF, Greenfield C, Chu CM, Karayiannis P, Dunk A, Lok ASF, Lai CL, Yeoh EK, Monjardino JP, Wankya BM, Thomas HC (1986) Integration of HBV-DNA may not be a prerequisite for the maintenance of the state of malignant transformation. Hepatol 2:218–229
Gerber MA, Thung SN (1985) Biology of disease. Molecular and cellular pathology of hepatitis B. Lab Invest 52:572–590
Goudeau A, Lo KJ, Coursaget P, Tong MJ, Yeh CL, Tsai YT, Lee JK, Wu TC, Yeh SH, Lee SD (1983) Prevention of hepatitis B virus infection in children born to HBsAg positive/HBeAg positive mothers. Preliminary results of active and passive-active immunization. Dev Biol Stand 54:399–404
Heermann KH, Goldmann U, Schwartz W, Seyfarth T, Baumgarten H, Gerlich WH (1984) Large surface proteins of hepatitis B virus containing the pre-S sequence. J Virol 52:396–402
Hilleman MR (1985) Newer directions in vaccine development and utilization. J Inf Dis 151:407–419
Hilleman MR, Bertland AU, Buynak EB, Lampson GP, McAleer WJ, McLean AA, Roehm RR, Tytell AA (1978) Clinical and laboratory studies of HBsAg vaccine. In: Vyas GN, Cohen SN, Schmid R (eds) Viral hepatitis. Franklin Institute, Philadelphia, pp 525–538
Hilleman MR, Bynak EB, Markus HZ, Maigetter RZ, McAleer WJ, McLean AA, Miller WJ, Wampler DE, Weibel RE (1984) Control of hepatitis B virus infection: vaccines produced from Alexander cell line and from recombinant yeast cell cultures. In: Vyas GN, Dienstag JL, Hoofnagle JH (eds) Viral hepatitis and liver disease. Grune and Stratton, Orlando, pp 307–314
Hummel M, Thorley-Lawson DA, Kieff E (1984) An Epstein-Barr virus DNA fragment encodes messages for the two major envelope glycoproteins (gp350/300 and gp 220/200). J Virol 49:413–417
Infectious Diseases Society (1986) Acquired immunodeficiency syndrome. J Inf Dis 154:1–9
Jameel S, Siddiqui A (1986) The human hepatitis B virus enhancer requires *trans*-acting cellular factor(s) for activity. Mol Cell Biol 6:710–715
Kanai K, Takehiro A, Noto H, Nishida M, Takahashi K, Kawashima Y, Igarashi Y, Matsushita K, Shimizu M (1985) Prevention of perinatal transmission of hepatitis B virus (HBV) to children of e antigen-positive HBV carrier mothers by hepatitis B immune globulin and HBV vaccine. J Inf Dis 151:287–290
Klein G (ed) (1980) Viral oncology. Raven, New York
Klinkert MQ, Theilmann L, Pfaff E, Schaller H (1986) Pre-s_1 antigens and antibodies early in the course of acute hepatitis B virus infection. J Virol 58:522–525
Lo KJ, Tsai YT, Lee SD, Wu TC, Wang JW, Chen GH, Yeh CL, Chiang BN, Yeh SH, Goudeau A, Coursaget P, Tong MJ (1985) Immunoprophylaxis of infection with hepatitis B virus in infants born to hepatitis B surface antigen-positive carrier mothers. J Inf Dis 152:817–822
McAleer WJ, Buynak EB, Maigetter RZ, Wampler DE, Miller WJ, Hilleman (1984) Human hepatitis B vaccine from recombinant yeast. Nature 307:178–180

Milich DR, Thornton GB, Neurath AR, Kent SB, Michel ML, Tiollais P, Chisari FV (1985) Enhanced immunogenicity of the pre-S region of hepatitis B surface antigen. Science 228:1195–1199

Morgan AJ, Smith AR, Barker RN, Epstein MA (1984) A structural investigation of the Epstein-Barr (EB) virus membrane antigen glycoprotein, pg 340. J Gen Virol 65:397–404

Moss B, Smith GL, Gerin JL, Purcell RH (1984) Use of vaccinia virus as a vector for the construction of live recombinant hepatitis B virus vaccines. In: Vyas GN, Dienstag JL, Hoofnagle JH (eds) Viral hepatitis and liver disease. Grune and Stratton, Orlando, pp 293–306

Nethersell A, Sikora K (1985) Interferons and malignant disease. In: Taylor-Papadimitriou J (ed) Interferons. Their impact in biology and medicine. Oxford University Press, Oxford, pp 127–145

Neurath AR, Kent SBH, Strick N, Taylor P, Stevens CE (1985) Hepatitis B virus contains pre-S gene-encoded domains. Nature 315:154–156

Newman MJ, Baker IT, Reitz MS, Eiden M, Blattner WA, Gallo RC, Manns DL (1986) Serological characterization of human T-cell leukemia (lymphotropic) virus, type I (HTLV-I) small envelope protein. Virology 150:106–116

Offensperger W, Wahl S, Neurath AR, Price P, Strick N, Kent SBH, Christman JK, Acs G (1985) Expression in *Escherichia coli* of a cloned DNA sequence encoding the pre-S region of hepatitis B virus. Proc Natl Acad Sci USA 82:7540–7544

Purcell RH, Gerin JL (1985) Prospects for second and third generation hepatitis B vaccines. Hepatology 5:159–163

Rasheed S, Norman GL, Gill PS, Meyer PR, Cheng L, Levine AM (1986) Virus-neutralizing activity, serologic heterogeneity, and retrovirus isolation from homosexual men in the Los Angeles area. Virology 1500:1–9

Robinson WS, Miller RH, Klote L, Marion PL, Lee SC 61984) Hepatitis B virus and hepatocellular carcinoma. In: Vyas GN, Dienstag JL, Hoofnagle JH (eds) Viral hepatitis and liver disease. Grune and Stratton, Orlando, pp 245–263

Sarma PS, Gruber J (1986) Meeting highlights. Vaccination approaches for retrovirus infection. JNCI 76:769–777

Scolnick EM, McLean AA, West DJ, Dienstag JL, Watkins E, Deinhardt F, Jilg W (1984) Antibody and clinical responses among healthy adults to a hepatitis B vaccine made by recombinant DNA. In: Vyas GN, Dienstag JL, Hoofnagle JH (eds) Viral hepatitis and liver disease. Grune and Stratton, Orlando, pp 315–317

Seeger C, Ganem D, Varmus HE (1986) Biochemical and genetic evidence for the hepatitis B virus replication strategy. Science 232:477–484

Starcich, Hahn BH, Shaw GM, McNeely PD, Modrow S, Wolf H, Parks ES, Parks WP, Josephs SF, Gallo RC, Wong-Staal F (1986) Identification and characterization of conserved and variable regions in the envelope gene of HTLV-III/LAV, the retrovirus of AIDS. Cell 45:637–648

Stevens CE, Taylor PE, Tong MJ, Toy PT, Vyas GN (1984) Hepatitis B vaccine: an overview. In: Vyas GN, Dienstag JL, Hoofnagle JH (eds) Viral hepatitis and liver disease. Grune and Stratton, Orlando, pp 275–291

WHO Collaborating Centres on AIDS: Memorandum from a WHO meeting (1986). Bull WHO 64: 37–46

Zachoval R, Jilg W, Lorbeer B, Schmidt M, Deinhardt F (1984) Passive/active immunization against hepatitis B. J Inf Dis 150:112–117

Zanetti AR, Dentico P, Del Vecchio Blanco C, Sagnelli E, Villa E, Ferroni P, Bergamini F (1986) Multicenter trial on the efficacy of HBIG and vaccine in preventing perinatal hepatitis B. Final report. J Med Virol 18:327–334

Zuckermann AJ (1985) New hepatitis B vaccines. Br Med J 290:492–496

Summary of Discussion: Session 5

G. Hunsmann

The question was raised whether the presence of papovavirus (HPV) genomes in over 80% of cervical cancer biopsy specimens could be explained by the fact that these carcinoma cells are particularly good hosts for HPV. Dr zur Hausen answered that at least in the human system it is very difficult to define tumor cells that are transformed by mechanisms other than viruses. He than referred to a recent publication by Cori showing that mice transgenic for a modified myc gene expressed this gene, whereby the normal alleles are surpressed. Under these conditions the cells continuously grow and poliferate, yet they are not malignant. After a longer period of time, monoclonal tumors appear in the mice. This shows that expression of this oncogene is clearly not sufficient for malignant transformation. A similar situation may exist in humans Burkitt's lymphoma. In this case a few percent of tumors do not contain Epstein-Barr virus (EBV) DNA. Nevertheless, EBV plays a role in malignant transformation, which we do not understand totally at the moment.

Another discussant asked whether the presence of viral genomes in the tumor cells is related to a particular pattern of oncogene expression. The data available at present are not conclusive. At least some cervical carcinomas contain an amplified myc gene and in these cells the integrational site of HPV is close to the myc gene. However, this situation might be related to tumor progression rather than to early events in tumor development.

It was asked whether after treatment of these patients with cervical carcinoma the HPV genome would still be present in cervical cells. Dr zur Hausen replied that his group has not had a chance yet to analyse this, but that it would be surprising not to find the virus in these patients. Several of these individuals already have premalignant lesions. Thus, he said he would anticipate that every patient maintains the HPV infection for life or at least a very long period of life. Dr zur Hausen then added that there is an interesting correlation between the degree of malignancy and certain HPV types found in the tumor. HPV16 is found in mild displasias rather rarely, while it is regularly present in moderate and severely altered cells, and also in a large number of cervical cancers. Furthermore, the expression of viral gene functions is obviously related to the transformed state. Therefore, it appears very likely that there is a causal relationship between these virus infections and cervical cancer.

How could the long latency period of cervical carcinoma after HPV infection be explained? Dr zur Hausen thinks that in addition to HPV infection there are two hits required in the cellular genome to inactivate the set of cellular genes, which control the virus infection. Such an explanation is consistent for the relatively shorter latency period of Burkitt's lymphoma, where only two events are needed, the translocation of the myc gene and the uptake of the virus.

Someone noted that in those areas of the Third World where an early infection with hepatitis B virus (HBV) takes place, a large number of persistent infections occur. This situation could be explained by immune defects in these people. Otherwise the virus would have been eliminated by the immune system. He than questioned whether the vaccine could work in this situation, where there is obviously a defect of the immune system. Dr. Deinhardt replied that the anti-HBV titers in the Chinese and African population are somewhat lower than those found in Europeans and North Americans. But on the other hand the immune response to a vaccine already applied in certain parts of China and Africa would be sufficient to block HBV infection.

How could the relatively long latency period for the development of hepatomas in woodchucks kept under experimental conditions be explained without implying external cofactors? Dr. Deinhardt replied that there was no identifiable reason other than the virus infection for the development of hepatomas in these animals.

Another discussant raised the point that in Scandinavia the ratio of infection with HBV of men and women is about equal, but that hepatocellular carcinoma is more frequently found in men. Dr. Deinhardt replied that alcohol consumption may be an additional factor for the development of hepatocellular carcinoma in Scandinavia. He then explained that only small parts of the viral genome were found in a certain fraction of tumor cells. Therefore, HBV is only one factor in the development of hepatocellular carcinoma. But in Taiwan the hepatocellular carcinoma developed 160 times more frequently in HBV-infected individuals than in uninfected matched controls.

It was asked whether results from studies on mouse hepatitis virus would be relevant for human hepatitis. Dr. Deinhardt explained that this virus does not belong to the hepatna virus group. Dr. zur Hausen stated that data from studies with mouse hepatitis virus for this reason cannot be transferred to men. Dr. Wecker added that in mice the major factor in determining the outcome of a virus infection, including those with tumor viruses, is a strain-specific response of the immune system. In this context Dr. Deinhardt remarked that Chinese immigrating to the United States have a lower risk of hepatocellular carcinoma. This is certainly not due to changes in the food habits, but rather to a change in the hygienic standard. Thus, the major determiner for the development of hepatocellular carcinoma after HBV infection seems to be infection early in life.

Summary of Round Table Discussion on Strategies Against Tobacco Cancer

G. EISENBRAND

Participants: M. Franke, D. Henschler (Chairman), D. Hoffmann, D. Schmähl, C. Straub-Blum, K. Thurau, I. Vogt-Moykopf, E. L. Wynder

At the beginning the long-lasting stagnation concerning improvements in the treatment of bronchial cancer was stressed. Now, as before, there have been few successful long-term effects (10%). Tobacco-induced cancer is to be overcome mostly by prevention. The discussion therefore concentrated on the possibilities of primary prevention. The following points were discussed in some detail.

What can be achieved by health education and education programs? Dr. Wynder explained a program which is planned in eight towns in the USA over the next 7 years, called the "Community Education Program." It is financed by the National Cancer Institute (NCI) and has considerable support from individuals. Childrens' education is one of the focal issues: the young school child will be instructed about the constitution and biological functioning of his body and the value of health through illustrative material and health checklists. At the same time there will be intensive education of parents, relatives, and teachers (peer groups). The example of these groups of people has proven to be significant to someone who is deciding whether to become a smoker or nonsmoker.

Programs with the same objective are being offered in Germany by government institutions. However, they are not to be compared with the American initiatives. Health education, it is true, is offered as an obligatory subject integrated with other subjects (biology, social education), but it is not taught in such a concentrated manner to the youngest pupils as a preventive measure.

Then were complaints about the massive advertising of smoking in the media. The efficacy of reducing advertisement has however been questioned somewhat by pointing to the high numbers of smokers in countries with little or no advertising. It is believed to be more effective and more promising to influence the attitudes or ways of acting of parents and relatives (peer persons) (Wynder).

The participants in the discussion agreed on the fact that learning/training of health consciousness and proper ways of acting cannot be the only preventive strategy. It is recognized that the best prevention is to stop smoking or to avoid starting smoking; there is a clear reduction of the risk of cancer among this group of persons.

Efforts to obtain a less harmful cigarette by reducing the tar content from the original 40 mg/cigarette to about 12–14 mg/cigarette should definitely be continued, according to prevailing opinion. A value of about 10 mg/cigarette of condensate and of 1 mg of nicotine should be aimed for. Even if this considerable reduction is partly undone by an increase in individual cigarette consumption, epidemiological data showing a reduction of cancer incidence after introduction of the "lighter" cigarette justify the concept of the less harmful cigarette. An additional measure is to reduce the nitrate content which has been raised during the past few years as more and more parts of plants are used that are rich in nitrate. Nitrate is one of the principal factors for the development of the highly carcinogenic nitrosocompounds in smoke (Hoffmann).

Further preventive measures concern passive smoking. The forbidding of smoking in public conveyances and indoor areas is a measure with considerable signal effects that could be particularly successful.

The discussion took place with the lively participation of the audience who made some essential contributions. One of the suggestions was to do away with the smoking rooms still existant at some schools. Teachers should be admonished to not smoke while at school. The considerable financial support for cultivating tobacco by the EEC was considered scandalous, especially with respect to the comparably tiny expenditure for research into the prevention of tobacco cancer.

Efforts to improve health education in Germany which are still unsatisfying must be intensified. The American example shows us that this is possible with appropriate application.

Subject Index

Batch number: 10704763

Printed by Printforce, the Netherlands